ETHICAL AND LEGAL ISSUES IN HOME HEALTH CARE

Case Studies and Analyses

AMY MARIE HADDAD, PhD, RN, C
Assistant Professor
School of Pharmacy and Allied Health Professions
Associate, Center for Health Policy and Ethics
Creighton University
Omaha, Nebraska

MARSHALL B. KAPP, JD, MPH
Professor
Department of Community Health
School of Medicine
Wright State University
Dayton, Ohio

APPLETON & LANGE
Norwalk, Connecticut/San Mateo, California

0-8385-2277-7

Notice: Our knowledge in clinical sciences is constantly changing. As new information becomes available, changes in treatment and in the use of drugs become necessary. The authors and the publisher of this volume have taken care to make certain that the doses of drugs and schedules of treatment are correct and compatible with the standards generally accepted at the time of publication. The reader is advised to consult carefully the instruction and information material included in the package insert of each drug or therapeutic agent before administration. This advice is especially important when using new or infrequently used drugs.

91 92 93 94 95 / 10 9 8 7 6 5 4 3 2 1

Prentice Hall International (UK) Limited, *London*
Prentice Hall of Australia Pty. Limited, *Sydney*
Prentice Hall Canada Inc., *Toronto*
Prentice Hall Hispanoamericana, S.A., *Mexico*
Prentice Hall of India Private Limited, *New Delhi*
Prentice Hall of Japan, Inc., *Tokyo*
Simon & Schuster Asia Pte. Ltd., *Singapore*
Editora Prentice Hall do Brasil, Ltda., *Rio de Janeiro*
Prentice Hall, *Englewood Cliffs, New Jersey*

Library of Congress Cataloging-in-Publication Data

Haddad, Amy Marie.
Ethical and legal issues in home health care / by Amy Marie Haddad, Marshall B. Kapp.
p. cm.
Includes bibliographical references.
ISBN 0-8385-2277-7
1. Home care services—Moral and ethical aspects. 2. Home care services—Law and legislation. I. Kapp, Marshall B. II. Title.
[DNLM: 1. Ethics, Medical. 2. Home Care Services. 3. Home Care Services—legislation. WY 115 H126e]
RA645.3.H32 1990
174′.2—dc20
DNLM/DLC 90-1016
for Library of Congress CIP

Acquisitions Editor: Marion Kalstein Welch
Production Editor: Jeff vonLiebermann
Designer: Janice Barsevich

PRINTED IN THE UNITED STATES OF AMERICA

Contributors

Amy Marie Haddad, PhD, RN, C
Assistant Professor
School of Pharmacy and Allied Health Professions
Associate, Center for Health Policy and Ethics
Creighton University
Omaha, Nebraska

Andrew Jameton, PhD
Associate Professor
Department of Preventive and Societal Medicine
University of Nebraska Medical Center
Omaha, Nebraska

Marshall B. Kapp, JD, MPH
Professor
Department of Community Health
School of Medicine
Wright State University
Dayton, Ohio

Steven S. Martin, RN, C
Director
Health Services Research
Blue Cross and Blue Shield of Nebraska
Omaha, Nebraska

Contents

Preface

A home care client refuses to comply with the plan of care, but still wants the nurses to visit. A ventilator-dependent client decides that he has had enough and wants the ventilator turned off. The parents of a chronically ill child are emotionally and physically exhausted, yet want to keep their child at home. These are the types of cases that frequently confront and perplex home care providers. Is it ethical? Is it legal? What is the right thing to do? We decided to write this book in order to help answer these commonly asked questions. Actual case studies are used to present ethical and legal issues in home health care. Though the majority of work in health care law and ethics has been in the acute care setting, home care requires a new perspective. This book provides that perspective with an appreciation of the unique environment in home care and its distinct challenges.

ORGANIZATION

Every clinical decision has legal and ethical underpinnings. In this litigious society, health care providers often first turn to the law to resolve practice dilemmas. It is the intent of this book to emphasize the complimentary, intricate relationship between law and ethics in light of the most common practice dilemmas encountered in home health care. The book begins with an overview of ethics terminology, decision making, and law.

Chapter 2 provides a historical backdrop for the present discussion in ethics in home care. The reader will be surprised and perhaps amused to find that many of the modern ethical problems in home care troubled their counterparts in the early 1900s. Some of the guidance and advice offered then is practical in today's dilemmas.

Chapter 3 focuses on the ethical conflicts at the most personal level of home care—the relationship between direct care providers and the client and family. The case of a ventilator-dependent client and her family is explored in depth. Chapter 4 examines a particularly troubling and contemporary issue—withholding and withdrawing life-sustaining treatment.

Chapter 5 considers some of the more pressing economic issues in home care such as restrictions on reimbursement, needy clients and lack of funding, and the disparity between reimbursement for products versus service. In Chapter 6, we turn to the regulatory issues that influence and structure home care practice, including licensure, certification, fraud and abuse, antitrust, and price discrimination. Chapter 7 focuses on the relationship between employer and employee and includes an exploration of the unique role of the home health aide and the ever-present concern regarding malpractice. Chapter 8 provides practical advice on the role of legal counsel in home care, and Chapter 9 explores the diversity of issues involving legal liability.

Wherever possible, specific cases have been used to illustrate potential legal problems and methods to avoid or minimize them. Finally, Chapter 10 examines organizational values, codes of ethics, and the role of ethics committees in home care.

Readers may or may not agree with our analyses of particular cases or issues, but if they begin the process of critically analyzing the issues presented by applying some of the methods we have proposed, the purpose of the book will have been fulfilled. This book is a starting point in the search for workable solutions to the myriad ethical and legal problems encountered in home care.

Amy Marie Haddad
Marshall B. Kapp

Chapter 1

Theoretical Bases for Ethics and Law

Amy Marie Haddad
Marshall B. Kapp

Case 1–1. A Question of Stealing
Case 1–2. Staffing and Staff Competency
Case 1–3. Use of Illegal Drugs
Case 1–4. The Appropriateness of Elder Care

Home health care, like every other area of the health care system in the past two decades, is changing and growing. Since the inception of Medicare in 1965, home care services have continually adapted and expanded to meet the needs of a changing population (Leader, 1986; Lerman, 1987). Since 1984, the advent of prospective pricing by Medicare and other third-party payers, combined with the increasing elderly population and other high-risk groups, and technological advances have shifted health care dollars to the home care sector. Home health care has become a safe, effective alternative to acute hospitalization or a stay in a skilled nursing facility.

All of the factors that have encouraged growth in home care have also bred novel and complex problems. There is ever-increasing competition for revenue with seemingly slimmer profit margins. Home care agencies—hospital, community or independents—go head-to-head with pharmacies, infusion therapy companies, and durable medical equipment suppliers for the same client. Competition has made it easy to forget the basic values of home care, which are to improve and maintain a client's quality of life (Lachman, 1988).

The elderly cohort has been most affected by the shift to prospective payment under Medicare, which has in turn affected home care. Problems in discharge and the need for home services are a major concern of families and their elderly members. Even though there is an obvious increase in the need for posthospital care, there has been limited adaptation of Medicare benefits to meet this need. Planning and providing care for the elderly has become more complex and more frustrating for home care providers.

Another potential problem area is the introduction of extremely complex clients to the home care setting. The complexity of care requires the involvement of numerous members of the health care team. Chances for conflict, fragmentation, breaches in confidentiality, and miscommunication increase as more people are involved in a client's care. For example, in the case of children with acquired immunodeficiency syndrome (AIDS), 4 to 15 community agencies may work with one family (Woodruff & Sterzin, 1988).

Complex clients require complex technology. The development of sophisticated technology and its use in the home have allowed many clients to return home who would not have been able to do so in the past. We seldom question if we have the technical capability to take a client home, but we increasingly ask what is in the best interest of the client and family? Should this particular technology be used? What are the stressors that will be introduced into the client's and family's lives by the use of this particular technology? When is it appropriate to remove or discontinue technological support in the home? These are ethical and legal questions, and the best clinical skills are of limited help in resolving them.

All of these factors: reimbursement, changes in demography, and technological advances have ethical and legal implications. Ethical and legal principles in home health care do not differ significantly from other areas of health care. All of the standard concerns in health care can be found here: professional competency, confidentiality, the rights or autonomy of the client, beneficence or the duty of the health care provider to help, price discrimination, kickbacks and fraud, termination of life-sustaining treatment, truth telling, fair reimbursement, and distribution of resources.

THE CONTEXT OF HOME CARE

Though the principles are the same as other areas of health care, the specific answers may not be. The context of home care requires new answers to the questions that are presented throughout this book. Since law and ethics often combine in decision making, it is appropriate to combine the two disciplines in this discussion about the most pressing problems in home care. The home care provider must consider moral duty and the requirements of law in making decisions about care delivery. In so doing, the home care provider must also keep in mind the prevailing standard of care. Only a few cases in home care need be discussed to illustrate the intricate relationship between ethics and law. Consider the following cases from home care practice:

Case 1–1. A Question of Stealing

Pat Jones is a new homemaker–home health aide. She has been assigned to care for Mrs. Clark, a frail, confused 90-year-old. Mrs. Clark is extremely wealthy and her twenty-four-hour care is privately paid for by a trust, as she has no immediate family. Pat is being oriented to the case by Bev Hines, who has been caring for Mrs. Clark for the last 4 years.

Pat stays with Mrs. Clark while Bev makes her weekly trip to the grocery store. When Bev returns from the store, Pat notices there is no change from the $20.00 Bev took from Mrs. Clark's weekly allowance, even though the total bill for the groceries was only $5.85. Pat musters the courage to ask Bev about this. Bev replies, "Oh, I always keep the change from shopping. No one ever asks for receipts for these little trips to the grocery store. She doesn't seem to miss it. Besides, what's ten or fifteen dollars to her? You're not going to say anything about this, are you?"

Case 1–2. Staffing and Staff Competency

A flu epidemic has hit four nurses on one of the most difficult ventilator cases that the We Care Home Care Agency manages. As Lindy Shepard, the nursing supervisor, scrambles to rearrange the schedules of her most skilled staff to cover the case, one more nurse on the case calls in sick. Now Lindy has a hole on the eleven-to-seven shift. She thinks that the evening nurse might stay until 1 AM and the day nurse could come in at 6 AM, but she doesn't know what to do about the hours from 1 AM to 6 AM. The only possible option is a newly hired nurse who has expressed a great deal of interest in ventilator care. Unfortunately, though she has completed the inservice training program on ventilator care, she has never taken care of a ventilator-dependent client. Should Lindy assign her and hope it's a quiet night? "After all," she reasons, "I'm just a phone call away. What could possibly go wrong?"

Case 1–3. Use of Illegal Drugs

Jill Walker is receiving chemotherapy in the home. One afternoon, the nurse arrives early to find Jill and her husband, Ted, sharing a pipe of what appears to be marijuana. Somewhat sheepishly, Ted explains, "This relaxes Jill so much and she doesn't get nauseated like she used to before we started smoking grass. She also has a better appetite." What Ted says is true. Jill has done much better with chemotherapy and has even gained some weight. The nurse wishes he hadn't seen this. Now what is he supposed to do?

Case 1–4. The Appropriateness of Elder Care

On a postpartum visit for a low-birth-weight infant, the nurse questions Mrs. Carey, the mother of four children, about the care of the newborn since her return home from the hospital. Mrs. Carey replies, "The baby's doing fine. Now I have more time to spend with her since I figured out how to take care of Grandpa."

The nurse questions further about Grandpa. "You see," Mrs. Carey explains, "I have to take care of my husband's dad. He's really goofy—wets the bed, wanders off, gets into all sorts of trouble. With the new baby and the other kids to watch, I couldn't be chasing him too. So I fixed a place for him in the basement." The nurse asks to see Grandpa and Mrs. Carey readily complies. After descending the steps to the basement, Mrs. Carey unlocks a door to approximately half of the basement. The room is clean and bare except for a plastic-covered mattress on the floor. Two windows let in some sunlight in addition to an overhead light. Grandpa is wandering aimlessly around the room and pays no attention to Mrs. Carey or the nurse. Grandpa is wearing only adult diapers and a long-sleeved shirt.

Mrs. Carey seems pleased and proud of her solution. "See," she says, "He can't run away, he can't fall out of bed, and I can keep him clean in the shower over there. He can still feed himself so I just bring down his meals." The nurse has never encountered anything quite like this. Should she involve adult protective services or not?

DISTINGUISHING BETWEEN ETHICS AND LAW

In each of the previously described cases, there are legal and ethical questions. At times it is difficult to distinguish where law ends and ethics begins or vice versa. Former Chief Justice of the Supreme Court Earl Warren described the relationship between ethics and law as follows:

> In civilized life, Law floats in a sea of Ethics. Each is indispensable to civilization. Without Law, we should be at the mercy of the least scrupulous; without Ethics, Law could not exist. Without ethical consciousness in most people, lawlessness would be rampant. Yet without Law, civilization could not exist, for there are always people who, in the conflict of human interest, ignore their responsibility to their fellowman (Warren, 1962, p. 2).

The relationship between ethics and law is intricate and delicate. One clear distinction, though, is in the enforceability of the obligation to follow the stated norm in both disciplines. "The obligation of the law usually involves a material penalty of one type or another, ie, a fine or a prison sentence. The obligation of ethics is one of conscience. Even though violating ethical norms may not involve material loss, one's integrity and authority are weakened or lost by violating ethical norms" (O'Rourke & Brodeur, 1989, p. 17).

An additional question often arises: which comes first—law or ethics? Law orders our social and institutional relationships and thus embodies ethical commitments. But it is too crude a measure of what is right to resolve complex ethical dilemmas. However, in home care practice, as in other areas of health care, we are more aware of the potential for legal liability than our moral responsibility. So we often turn to law first and ask, "Is it legal?" before considering the ethical implications in a case. Properly, laws should be founded on ethical norms. So, in each instance we should ask: "Is the issue in question one in which moral duty is involved? If yes, has this moral duty become a legal requirement of practice?" (Hamner, Scoggin, & White, 1981, p. 26).

Application to Clinical Actions

The following figure graphically illustrates the relationship between ethics and law in home-care-practice situations.

An example of an action that is both ethical and legal is the doctrine of informed consent (see Chapter 3). The legal development of the doctrine of informed consent has had a rather lengthy and tortuous route through various court cases. A landmark legal principle was established in 1914, when Judge Cardozo stated that "[e]very human being of adult years and sound mind has a right to determine what shall be done with his own body . . ." (Schloendorff v Society of New York Hospital, 211 NY 125, 129 [1914]).

This principle became the basis of contemporary discussions of informed consent. The doctrine became further refined by the ". . . development of a 'consumer's rights' orientation in society at large, "so that" judges in torts and contract cases beginning in the 1950s were increasingly willing to restrict the freedom of the party holding the upper hand in various settings usually the seller of the goods and services" (Capron, 1988, p. 39).

The most recent refinement of the doctrine has been the "reasonable man" standard. Instead of a community of physicians determining what information should be told to a client, a physician, in many states, is required to inform a client in terms of what a "reasonable man" would want to know (Mazur, 1986).

The ethical development of informed consent reflects the view that personal autonomy should be highly valued and respected. Therefore, informed consent is a concrete manifestation of an individual's right to self-determination and respect for preferences related to health care.

	ETHICAL	UNETHICAL
	Ethical and Legal	Unethical and Legal
LEGAL	Informed consent	Regulatory limitations on medicare visits
	Ethical and Illegal	Unethical and Illegal
ILLEGAL	Inaccurate record keeping in order to continue needed services	Abandonment

An example of a situation that is legal but often considered unethical is the regulatory limitation on Medicare home care visits. In order to qualify for Medicare home health care, ". . . a person must be confined to his or her residence (homebound), be "under a physician's care, and need part-time or intermittent skilled nursing care and/or physical or speech therapy. The services must be furnished under a plan of care prescribed and periodically reviewed by a physician" (Medicare Home Health Care, 1986, p. 11).

The limitations of the regulation might have been fair and adequate to meet the needs of Medicare beneficiaries in 1965 but are grossly inadequate today. The regulations have been periodically reinterpreted by the Health Care Financing Administration to the fiscal intermediaries who ultimately decide if reimbursement will be approved or denied. Home care providers have to contend with these new interpretations that generally narrow the window of eligibility. Yet, home care providers must deal with clients who are clearly in need. For example, consider the following case.

> Mr. Smith is a diabetic with an old CVA, whose caregiver wife is also ill and not able to participate in his care. His medical condition necessitates maximum assistance (two people) to get Mr. Smith up; he is incontinent and prone to skin breakdown and has a frequent

> history of pneumonia. Due to the combination of complex medical problems that his physician felt required the monitoring of an RN and the services of the home health aide, a plan of treatment was established by the physician that directed an RN to draw monthly blood sugars and monitor the diabetic condition in coordination with an intensive personal care plan involving bathing Mr. Smith three times a week, an exercise program, and observation of skin condition.
>
> Prior to the switch to a new regional intermediary, this case was considered as an acceptable level of medically reasonable and necessary care. However, Illinois reported that a dermatologist, who will remain nameless, told them that no elderly patient needed more than one bath per week and, subsequently, Mr. Smith's aide care was denied as not reasonable and necessary. (Davis & Pritchard-Pullins, 1987, p. 24)

Home care providers find this type of case frustrating and demoralizing. One method of dealing with the frustration is to choose an action that some believe is ethical but illegal, as in the case of technical fraud. For example, everyone involved in the rehabilitation of a stroke patient must submit reports to Medicare documenting the progress of the client. When no further progress can be shown, services are no longer reimbursed. However, ". . . progress does not occur at a consistent rate; rather it is marked by some periods of rapid improvement interspersed with other periods of almost no perceptible change (plateaus). Yet Medicare and other agencies make little or no allowance for these plateau periods and treatment is discontinued" (Purtilo & Cassel, 1981, p. 4).

The home care agency must decide between honestly reporting a client's lack of progress and losing coverage or lying to retain benefits for the client. There are ethical problems with this action, too, as deception breeds mistrust and erodes the integrity of those involved.

Finally, an action that is both illegal and unethical is abandonment. Abandonment is a type of actionable malpractice in which there is a unilateral severance by the physician of the physician–client relationship. It consists of a failure by the physician to continue to provide service without reasonable notice, at a time when there is still the necessity of continued medical attention (Louisell & Williams, 1989; McIntire, 1962). Though the development of abandonment as a separate and distinguishable category of malpractice litigation has been largely confined to medicine, the home care agency, as the direct provider of care, could be considered to be held to the same legal obligations to deliver care as the physician.

There is a legal and ethical obligation to continue care if the patient is in need of care and has no other recourse. Even if one is within legal rights to discontinue care (eg, the provider has made a reasonable but unsuccessful effort to transfer the client to a different provider), the ethical obligation remains to assist or render needed service, as that is the purpose of a profession: to subordinate personal feelings when professional services are needed (Bernzeig, 1981).

THE ELEMENTS OF ETHICS

Philosophy technically includes five fields of study: logic, the study of ideal methodology in thought and research; esthetics, the study of ideal form and beauty; politics, the study of ideal social organization; metaphysics, the study of the ultimate reality of things; and ethics (Durant, 1952). "Ethics is a disciplined study devoted to rational analysis and justification of moral principles which provides knowledge and insight regarding what we ought to do in order to attain the most of what is best in human life" (Chinn, 1979, p. *v*). The term *disciplined* refers to a process of organized reflection rather than intuition or responses at a "gut level." Justification refers to the reasons presented in an ethical deliberation for a specific action or actions that prove or demonstrate the action to be just, right, or valid.

The discipline of ethics studies human behavior and makes value judgments about what is good or bad and right or wrong. An ethics that prescribes what "ought" to be or ought to be done is often called a *normative* or *applied* ethics. Bioethics, or the study of ethics as applied to health care, is an example of normative ethics. The terms *ethics* and *morality* are often used interchangeably. Morals have been more specifically defined as ". . . a set of values or principles to which one is personally committed. Moral values or principles may be formal or informal, explicit or implicit" (Jameton, 1984, p. 5).

We face moral choices on a daily basis. We make choices in our personal and professional lives that reflect the complex value systems that we inherit from our families, religious backgrounds, education, and life experience. Even though we make ethical choices, it is a different and more difficult matter to explain how we arrived at our choice.

Ethical Principles

In making ethical decisions, principles and theories are used to guide the process. Principles are fundamental action guides specifying that some type of action is prohibited, required, or permitted in certain circumstances (Solomon, 1978). There are numerous ethical principles, but for the purposes of this book, several are introduced here and are explored in more detail throughout the remainder of this book.

Autonomy. The principle of autonomy requires that we respect individuals because they are human beings. This respect allows individuals freedom to form their own judgments and perform actions they choose. This means that individuals capable of doing so autonomously have the right to make their own choices about treatment or nontreatment (see Chapter 3).

The principle of respect for persons underlies ethical issues unique to home care such as informed consent in light of the often extended relationship between provider and client, family rules and expectations of providers, protection of privacy and confidentiality, the determination of competence and noncompliance.

Beneficence. The principle of beneficence reminds us of our duty to do good for others and to prevent harm. According to this principle, we are to refrain from harming others at all times (nonmaleficence) and to further the interests of others. The obligation of beneficence is dependent on the existence of a relationship (see Chapter 3).

The principle of beneficence includes the examination of the following concepts and issues: paternalism, distinguishing between dangerous and less-than-desirable care, the capabilities of an agency to provide safe and effective care for clients, discontinuing service and abandonment, and the moral obligations of the home care provider.

Justice. The two previously cited principles, autonomy and beneficence guide us in our interactions with one another. The principle of distributive justice moves the setting of ethical discussion to the level of the community. Distributive justice refers to the justified distribution of benefits and burdens in society. In claims of justice, we try to link persons to certain benefits and burdens that society can distribute (social goods), usually on the basis of some asset or characteristic of that person (Pinkard, 1986). Therefore, goods or services such as home care can be distributed based on the ability to pay, the health care needs or age of the person in question, or to those who would benefit the most from home care service. Since living in a community necessarily requires us to make claims against each other for available goods and services, justice provides the social rules that allow us to do this fairly.

The principle of justice requires that we examine the following issues: distribution of services, the appropriateness of home care, profit and loss, access to home care services, and levels of care.

Fidelity. The principle of fidelity, or faithfulness, includes obligations to be truthful and to keep promises (Ross, 1930). Making promises, implicitly or explicitly, and honoring them is an integral part of the health provider–client relationship. Fidelity is the foundation of trust. Fidelity "commits one to a reliability and constancy which is the formal fulfillment of faithfulness, that is, perseverance in one's promises" (Mitchell & Achtenberg, 1984, p. 18). The home care provider and its personnel often make promises to clients and families that prove to be impossible to keep because of restrictions in the number of available staff or reimbursement. These types of situations compromise fidelity.

A corollary principle, veracity, emphasizes the importance of honesty in a relationship. Telling the truth is recognized as a means to foster mutual respect and trust in the professional–client relationship. Arguments against honesty center around the need to protect the client from information that might be upsetting or emotionally harmful. This view always gives beneficence priority over veracity. However, ". . . if the health professional, both verbally and through his or her actions, conveys the message that he or she still cares, and has the intention and ability to comfort, then it is possible to tell the truth and still maintain the patient's trust and hope" (Purtilo & Cassel, 1981, pp. 74–75).

Normative Ethical Theories

Moral principles can often be in conflict and we are torn as to which principle takes priority over another. It is at this point that we move to the level of ethical theories to assist us in resolving the conflict. Ethical theories systematize and establish priorities among the principles previously mentioned and work out the details of their application to problems in home care and other areas of health care. There are several ethical theories but each ". . . represents a serious effort to supply a set of moral principles that are mutually consistent, in keeping with the facts of the world, and adequate for resolving moral difficulties" (Munson, 1983, p. 7).

Modern ethical theory has come to be classified into two major approaches: deontological and utilitarian. For the purposes of this book, an overview of the distinguishing features of the major theories will suffice in order to understand their application to the selected problems presented and, by extension, to actual problems encountered in daily practice. The reader is directed to the literature in the bibliography for further reference.

Deontological Theory. Deontologists argue that acts should be judged morally right or wrong because of qualities inherent in the act itself, and not primarily because of the good or bad outcomes of an action. (The Greek word *deon*, or binding duty, is the source of the term.) Deontologists judge the rightness of an act insofar as it fulfills some principle of duty. These types of theories are often referred to as "duty-based" theories.

Deontologists believe that our duties to others are manifold and diverse, some springing from special relationships. These relationships include that between a health professional and client, parent and child, and an employer and employee. These relationships have moral worth and should be considered when making an ethical decision.

Past actions or the history of our relationships also have moral meaning, according to deontologists. The principle of fidelity figures prominently in deontological theories. A moral commitment to keep a promise or fulfill an action creates an obligation beyond the usual respect due to persons and existing relationships.

Utilitarianism. According to the theory of utilitarianism, which can take many forms, no actions are good or evil in themselves; an action is good or morally right if it results in the most good possible in a given situation. Utilitarianism requires us to act so as to produce the greatest possible good-to-evil ratio for all concerned. If it is not possible to bring about good, then one is required to choose that action which brings about the least amount of evil or unhappiness.

Utilitarians see moral rules as a means to the fulfillment of individual needs as well as to the achievement of broad social goals, that is, to promote human welfare by minimizing harms and maximizing benefits (Beauchamp & Walters, 1982). Utilitarian theories are very popular in our society because they minimize self-interest by their emphasis on aggregate happiness and they allow flexibility in ethical decision.

Both major types of normative ethical theories have an appeal because of their consistency with our own value systems, their simplicity, or their usefulness in making ordinary, everyday ethical choices. In fact, the differences of the theories may not be as drastic as they appear in outline. It is possible for forms of utiliarianism and deontology to lead to identical rules and actions (Beauchamp & Childress, 1983).

However the choice regarding which theory to use in resolving a specific ethical dilemma is not arbitrary. Each theory commits us to different principles and priorities. The challenge is to apply a defensible argument for the alternatives we select, which is an integral step in ethical decision making.

Ethical Decision Making

Everyone involved in home care is involved in making ethical decisions. The process of decision making, choosing from among alternatives, can occur at a variety of levels—from a supervisor and a homemaker–home health aide discussing a case to an ethics committee (see Chapter 10)—and degrees of formality—from a specific judgment regarding the care of one client to policy development that will effect numerous clients.

Realistically, much of the decision making regarding daily practice occurs on an individual basis by those closest to the clients and their families. It is not always possible or necessary to formally consult an ethicist or ethics committee before making an ethical choice. Regardless of whether it is a solo or group effort, decision making requires critical thinking and should result in the choice of a morally justifiable action to be taken in a given situation (Thompson & Thompson, 1985).

Three prerequisites to effective decision making have been proposed: (1) we have to acknowledge that all choices are risky, which keeps us from choosing only those things that are comfortable or familiar; (2) we have to believe that there may be a better choice that is not so obvious, so we take the time to search for alternatives; and (3) we need to set aside sufficient time to look for the best alternative (Janis & Mann, 1977).

Given these prerequisites, there follows a five-step model for ethical decision making that will assist the home care professional in verifying that an ethical problem exists, and in choosing a justifiable course of action. This systematic approach can be applied to various types of practice dilemmas and allows for differences in values and clinical advances that necessarily change. The five steps are as follows:

- Respond to the "sense" or feeling something is wrong.
- Gather information.
- Identify the ethical problem.
- Seek a resolution.
- Work with others to determine action.

The five-step model will be applied to Pat Jones' dilemma in the first case study presented in this chapter to illustrate the process of decision making.

Respond to the "Sense" or Feeling Something Is Wrong. Though it has just been emphasized that ethical decision making is a logical, rational process, the first step is not. The first step is to respond to one's intuition that something is wrong in a given situation. Unlike noticeable signs and symptoms such as a rise in temperature or ecchymosis, there are no objective signs that one is involved in an ethical dilemma. Some of the most common warning signs that an ethical dilemma is in progress are: ". . . stress and tension intrapersonally or interpersonally; ineffective communication patterns such as avoidance, nagging, or silence; heightened emotional sensitivity with the feeling of self-doubt and the awareness of being trapped" (Salladay, 1986, p. 16).

In the case of Pat Jones, the new homemaker–home health aide responded to the feeling that something wasn't right regarding her coworker's action. Pat had to "muster the courage" to ask her coworker about keeping the change so there is evidence of some psychological conflict. However, Pat had the moral sensitivity to quickly move to the next step: gather information.

Gather Information. In order to make an informed decision, one must have the facts. It is important to ascertain the relevant facts in a given situation, those facts that impact on an ethical decision. By gathering the relevant facts, it is possible to determine if there is an ethical problem in the first place.

Generally speaking, the facts fall into two categories: clinical and situational. Clinical information includes all pertinent data related to diagnosis, prognosis, and treatment. As clinical ambiguity increases so do ethical tensions. Situational information includes background data on the people involved in a situation, their authority, values, and views; verbal and nonverbal communication; the setting and time; and the relationships of those involved.

When gathering information, many questions arise. In Mrs. Clark's case, Pat Jones might have wondered about the following questions: (1) What is going on here? (2) Is Bev stealing? (3) Does everyone on this case do this? (4) Does the home care agency know? (5) Does Mrs. Clark know? (6) Do the trustees at the bank that manage Mrs. Clark's trust know? (7) Should I say something? (8) If I say something, whom should I tell? (9) If I say something, will I get into trouble?

Pat knows that "keeping the change" has been going on for quite a while. At this juncture, she does not know if Bev is the only one involved. Pat does know that she is new to the home care agency and is therefore highly dependent on her coworkers for support and information.

The most important method of gathering relevant information is to listen and observe. The process of reflection and questioning will also help identify the focus of the "feelings" that triggered the response in the first place (Purtilo & Cassel, 1981). What was it that made Pat react? Was it Mrs. Clark's helplessness? Her coworker's callous response? A basic value that prohibits stealing?

Identify the Ethical Problem. Once the facts are clearly outlined, one can examine them to see whether it has the characteristics of an ethical problem: it does not belong solely within science, it is perplexing, and the answer has implications that touch many areas of human concern (Curtin, 1982). Because it deals with a wide range of imperatives and obligations of human dignity and conduct, ethics can serve as a guideline to identify the type of ethical problem in a specific case. It is also helpful to identify the ethical principles germane to the case.

Clearly, there is a legal problem in the case: stealing. It is against the law to steal. It is also unethical to steal, based on the principle of respect for persons. Mrs. Clark is a person and is therefore worthy of respect. Perhaps she is even more worthy of respect because she is frail, vulnerable, and dependent on others to look out for her well-being. The principle of beneficence also comes into play in this case. Though Bev argues that "She doesn't seem to miss it. Besides, what's ten or fifteen dollars to her?", the argument is not compelling. Indeed, Mrs. Clark may not miss the money and may even be able to afford to lose a little money each week. The fact that Mrs. Clark is wealthy does not justify Bev's action. Bev is certainly not helping Mrs. Clark by stealing from her, even though the harm may appear minimal. The principle of beneficence requires that not only should we refrain from harming others but that we help others further their legitimate interests.

Is there a conflict of obligations in the case? Pat Jones is obligated to care for Mrs. Clark, but she also has obligations to her coworkers, to her employer, and to herself. Which obligations take priority? Even if Pat chooses not to steal herself, she is still faced with the issue of complicity in wrongdoing. As in many cases, there are several ethical problems at work in the case.

Seek a Resolution. At this point, Pat should begin to explore possible courses of action. This is, indeed, the working phase of the decision-making process, and many individuals shy away from the task. "In order to reduce the stress of decision making, the fear of the unknown, and the threat of real or imaginary deadline, people often settle for the first available option, the safe choice, or the majority opinion" (Salladay, 1986, p. 26).

There are at least three courses of action available to Pat: (1) do nothing; (2) participate in stealing from Mrs. Clark; or (3) report her observations to her supervisor. In order to determine which options are morally justifiable, one must project probable consequences of each action and the underlying intention of the action. This process involves the application of the ethical theories and principles presented in this chapter. By following this process, some actions can be immediately rejected because they would result in harm or are in conflict with another basic ethical principle or personal value system.

If Pat uses a deontological theory to resolve her dilemma she would disapprove of Bev's action as incompatible with the respect, dignity, and equality that all human beings deserve. A deontologist would condemn stealing as injuring individuals and groups, as well as insulting the individual's basic right to fair and equal treatment. The action of stealing uses Mrs. Clark as a means to an end, which is unacceptable in a deontological framework. According to this line of reasoning, Bev's action is immoral and Pat has an obligation to report her observations to her supervisor.

If Pat were to take a utilitarian stance, she would not support an unqualified position on stealing. If stealing would be likely to produce more social good than any other alternative, then it would be good and right. If not, then it would be bad and wrong. The utilitarian theory is based on social utility and not on any inherent characteristic of the act itself. In order for Pat to decide if Bev's action is right or wrong, she would have to consider the effects of the alternatives facing her on everyone concerned. If she doesn't inform her supervisor of Bev's action, Mrs. Clark will continue to be victimized, Bev will profit, and Pat will be a co-conspirator in stealing. If she does inform her supervisor, Mrs. Clark will not continue to lose money, Bev may suffer the loss of her job or at least a reprimand, and Pat may not be accepted by her coworkers. In addition, Pat must calculate other consequences, such as the possibility of the trustees at the bank finding out, another coworker reporting the incident, and the ripple effects of each alternative. Pat would have to choose that action that would be likely to produce the most good for the most people concerned. Unlike the deontological perspective, utilitarianism could apparently endorse stealing in certain circumstances.

A resolution is sought, as opposed to a single solution. This distinction leaves the process open to renegotiation. It also encourages actually making a choice rather than searching endlessly for the "right" answer.

Work With Others to Determine a Course of Action. No one makes clinical decisions in a vacuum. The same is true for ethical decisions. Ethical problems are more likely to be resolved and fair decisions reached if the individuals involved have the opportunity to air their perceptions, values, and concerns. Group process can enrich decision making by providing a variety of options that would not be as apparent to an individual tackling the problem alone. Also, the group provides support and validates the ethical norms of the home care agency as a whole. It is appropriate for Pat to discuss her observations and concerns with her immediate supervisor. Together they can decide what to do.

Although moral issues may begin as vague perceptions, it has been demonstrated that through systematic reflection they can become more clearly articulated. Like ethics, law is a body of principles that regulates conflicting interests. Law, however, is much more tangible and usually clearer regarding what is permissible or not. At this juncture, we will cross the line between ethics and law to examine the origins of law and the practical application of the law to home care.

TYPES OF LAW

Law refers to human-made rules that regulate human social conduct in a formally perscribed and legally binding manner (Bernzeig, 1981, p. 3). Home care practice is affected by various types of law, which can be classified as follows:

Constitutional Law

"Constitutional law refers to the general organization, plan, and principles of a government. It is organic law, subject to amendment, that is made by the people as a whole. In this country the federal, state, and local governments all have written constitutions" (Kapp & Bigot, 1985, p. 8). A constitution grants legislative bodies the authority to enact different types of general laws.

Statutory Law

Statutory law is derived from formal legislative enactments. Laws passed by state legislatures or Congress are examples of statutory law. Laws established through legislation involve compromise. It is impossible for a legislative body to enact rules that comprehensively cover all types of human conduct in all situations.

Administrative Law

A type of law particularly applicable to home care practice is administrative law. "Administrative laws are called rules, regulations, or orders. They are enacted by administrative (executive) agencies, such as departments of health or public welfare, pursuant to powers delegated by the legislature" (Kapp & Bigot, 1985, p. 8). The Medicare and Medicaid regulations that have been enacted at the federal and state levels to implement home care statutes are examples of administrative laws. Rules and regulations have the full force of law behind them and, just like statutes, must be written, published, limited to future effect, addressed to all or a few, and consistent with the constitution (as well as the authorizing statute) (Kapp & Bigot, 1985, p. 8–9). Administrative law also includes judicial decisions about the meaning and effect of rules and regulations.

Common Law

Common law is the result of judicial decisions that interpret legal questions raised in disputes taken to court. This judge-made law is referred to as common law or case law to distinguish it from the laws passed by legislative enactments.

> For centuries, judges have built up a code of case law, and principles have been created and developed which, in the main, tend to keep abreast with, or generally just a little way behind, the changing social scene. It seems generally acceptable for judges, in some areas of law, though they are not elected representatives of the people, to make or develop new law. But in other areas there is considerable opposition to judges arrogating unto themselves the role of legislators. What is not clear is the kind of role the judges should adopt in relation to medical ethics. (Dworkin, 1988, p. 26)
> (Copyright 1988 by the Annals of the New York Academy of Sciences, New York. Reprinted with permission.)

Though the role of the judge is not clear in ethical decisions, it appears that resort to the courts is becoming a popular method for resolving ethical problems. "There has grown up an essentially lazy preference for litigation rather than legislation as the instrument of social change. Courts, you see, are quicker than legislatures, and so much tidier" (Will, 1986, p. 7).

Law can further be distinguished by classifying it as civil and criminal law. Criminal law relates solely to conduct that is considered an offense against the general public because it is detrimental to the welfare of society. Civil law is concerned with the legal rights and relationships that exist between private persons (Bernzweig, 1981). Liability for malpractice falls under the general classification of civil law (see Chapter 9).

Law contributes to a careful and cautious consideration of relevant issues and perspectives and asks questions that would not otherwise be asked (Kapp & Lo, 1986).

SUMMARY

Laws and the legal system help order society and, by extension, the health care system of which home care is a part. However, they are by no means the only element that helps us develop conduct that is socially and professionally acceptable. Ethics and professional values must also enter into the calculus if we are to have an environment that encourages the provision of humane, quality health care services.

The imprecise but real distinction between law and ethics has been drawn to illustrate that laws are helpful if they express sound ethical standards but should not be the sole basis for decision making. The select components of ethics and law were outlined to provide the tools to examine and analyze the more salient issues in home care that will be discussed in greater detail in subsequent chapters.

Staff members of home care agencies are involved in making ethical decisions on a daily basis. There are neither the time nor the resources to consult an expert in ethics every time a decision is made. Therefore, every staff member should possess the skills to sort through the ethical factors in a case and arrive at a justifiable resolution. This chapter offers a five-step model for ethical decision making that can be applied to many different types of dilemmas in home care practice.

REFERENCES

Beauchamp, T., & Childress, J.F. (1983). *Principles of Biomedical Ethics*. New York: Oxford University Press.

Beauchamp, T., & Walters, L. (1982). *Contemporary Issues in Bioethics* (2nd ed.). Belmont, Calif: Wadsworth Publishing Company.

Bernzeig, E.P. (1981). *The Nurse's Liability for Malpractice*. New York: McGraw Hill Book Company.

Capron, A.M. (1988). Harmonies and conflicts in law and biomedical ethics. *Annals of New York Academy of Sciences, 530*(June 15):37–45.

Chinn, P. (1979). From the editor. *Advances in Nursing Science, 1*(3): *v.*

Curtin, L. (1982). No rush to judgement. In L. Curtin & M.J. Flaherty (Eds.), *Nursing Ethics: Theories and Pragmatics* (pp. 57–66). Bowie, Md: Robert J. Brady Company.

Davis, E.J., & Pritchard-Pullins, M.L. (1987). The Medicare home care benefit today: The provider perspective. *PRIDE Institute Journal of Long Term Home Care, 6*(4):19–25.

Durant, W. (1952). *The Story of Philosophy*. New York: Washington Square Press.

Dworkin, G. (1988). The delicate balance: Ethics, law and medicine. *Annals New York Academy of Sciences, 530*(June 15):24–36.

Hamner, M.E., Scoggin, J.A., & White, B.D. (1981). The basis for ethico-legal instruction in the pharmacy curriculum. *American Journal of Pharmaceutical Education, 45*(1):25–29.

Jameton, A. (1984). *Nursing Practice: The Ethical Issues*. Englewood Cliffs, NJ: Prentice–Hall, Inc.

Janis, I.L., & Mann, L. (1977). *Decision Making: A Psychological Analysis of Conflict, Choice, and Commitment*. New York: The Free Press.

Kapp, M.B., & Bigot, A. (1985). *Geriatrics and the Law*. New York: Springer Publishing Company.

Kapp, M.B., & Lo, B. (1986). Legal perceptions and medical decision making. *The Milbank Quarterly, 64*(Suppl. 2): 163–202.

Lachman, B.G. (1988). Ethical issues in home health care. *The Consultant Pharmacist, 3*(1):32, 40–42, 44–45.

Leader, S. (1986). *Home health benefits under Medicare: A working paper*. Working paper prepared for the Public Policy Institute of the American Association of Retired Persons, Washington, DC.

Lerman, D. (1987). The home care opportunity. In D. Lerman (Ed.), *Home Care: Positioning the Hospital for the Future.* Chicago: American Hospital Publishing, Inc.

Louisell, D.W., & Williams, D. (1989). *Medical Malpractice* (Vol. 1). New York: Matthew Pender & Company, Inc.

Mazur, D.J. (1986). What should patients be told prior to a medical procedure? *The American Journal of Medicine, 81*(6):1051–1054.

McIntire, L.L. (1962). The action of abandonment in medical malpractice litigation. *Tulane Law Review, 34*:834–842.

Medicare Home Health Care. (1986). *Medicare: Need to Strengthen Home Health Care Payment Controls and Address Unmet Needs* (GAO/HRD 87–9). Washington, DC: US Government Printing Office.

Mitchell, C., & Achtenberg, B. (1984). *Code Gray: Study Guide.* Boston: Fanlight Productions.

Munson, R. (1983). *Intervention and Reflection: Basic Issues in Medical Ethics.* Belmont, Calif: Wadsworth Publishing Company.

O'Rourke, K., & Brodeur, D. (1989). *Medical Ethics: Common Ground for Understanding* (Vol. 2). St. Louis: The Catholic Health Corporation.

Pinkard, T. (1986, June). *Justice.* Paper presented at the Kennedy Institute of Ethics, Intensive Bioethics Course, Washington, DC.

Purtilo, R., & Cassel, C.K. (1981). *Ethical Dimensions in the Health Professions.* Philadelphia: W.B. Saunders Company.

Ross, W.D. (1930). *The Right and the Good.* New York: Oxford University Press.

Salladay, S. (1986). Ethical responsibility in mental health practice. In D.K. Kentsmith, S.A. Salladay, & P.A. Miya (Eds.), *Ethics in Mental Health Practice* (pp. 13–30). Orlando, Fla: Grune & Stratton, Inc.

Schloendorff v Society of New York Hospital, 211 NY 125, 129 (1914).

Solomon, W.D. (1978). Rules and principles. In W. T. Reich (Ed.), *Encyclopedia of Bioethics* (pp. 407–413). New York: The Free Press.

Thompson, J.E., & Thompson, H.O. (1985). *Bioethical Decision Making for Nurses.* Norwalk, Conn: Appleton-Century-Crofts.

Warren, E. (1962, November). Special address to the Lewis Marshall Award Dinner of the Jewish Theological Seminary of America, New York.

Will, G.F. (1986). For the handicapped, rights but no welcome. *Hastings Center Report, 16*(3):5–8.

Woodruff, G., & Sterzin, E.D. (1988). The transagency approach: A model for serving children with HIV infection and their families. *Children Today, 17*(3):9–11.

Chapter 2

Propriety and Tragedy: A Brief History of Ethics in Home Care

Andrew Jameton

This chapter provides a brief sketch of the history of nursing ethics in home care. It will not deal at all with the ancient history of nursing ethics before the first period of professionalization of nursing in the last half of the nineteenth century, even though most nursing work prior to the advent of hospitals was home care nursing. In the last century, nursing ethics can be divided roughly into three periods.

1. An "early" period from about 1890 to about 1939 when ethical concerns were prominent in the nursing literature and the major modes of nursing practice were private duty and visiting nursing in the home.
2. A "scientific" period from about 1939 to about 1977 when the terms "ethics" and "morality" practically disappeared from the

nursing literature despite the adoption in 1950 of the American Nurses' Association's first Code for Professional Nurses. During this period, ethical issues tended to be treated under such headings as "professional adjustments," "human relations," and similar psychological and sociological concepts (Densford & Everett, 1947; Spalding, 1939).

3. A "recent" period since 1977 marked by a renaissance of scholarship on ethics broadened by participation of philosophers, lawyers, and other non-nurses in major debates over ethics in patient care, in the uses of health care technology, and in access to care.

The focus of this chapter will primarily rest on the early phase of nursing ethics, because it set the tone and problems for the rest of the century, because it produced a rich variety of material, and because it provides striking contrasts to current approaches to ethics.

THE MAIN ISSUES

An important question occurs both in the history of ethics and in the anthropology of ethics: Are there universal moral principles that apply to all times and cultures? Identifying common practices among cultures, such as rules against murder or incest, tends to point toward universal constancies in ethics; finding divergent practices, such as varying rules governing kinship, private property, and religion, tends to suggest that there are no universals in ethics, or if there are, they are so distant from daily life as to be of little use in governing conduct.

Analogous to investigating varying cultures, it is also possible to travel in time to compare moral practices. By moving into the past, we can encounter our own culture in different guises. Do moral convictions change over time? More specifically, are professional moral traditions substantially the same and constant during the last century of nursing history, or do practices and concerns change radically so that the nursing ethics of a nurse visiting a home in the 1890s is substantially different from that of a nurse entering the home in the 1990s?

Differences and Similarities

As one might expect to find with polar contrasts, nursing ethics experienced a mix of constancies and change during the last century of its history. To consider notable points of change, the relationship of the nurse in the home to the servants in the home is not now so vital a question as it was for nurses in the early part of the century. Similarly, nurses in the 1990s must deal with providing technically complex care in the home, not as much of an issue in 1890. Also, nurses who wrote about ethics at the turn of the century tended to use different referents in their moral arguments. They were then inclined more often to refer to the Golden Rule, to the model of Christ, and to the reputation and character of the nurse than commentators on ethics do now. In the 1990s, the language of utilitarianism, patient autonomy, beneficence, and justice tend to occur more often.

We will discuss these changes in more detail below. Note here, however, that these changes raise questions about the foundations of ethics. Do these changes simply reflect changes in family, household, and technology, so that the same old moral principles are being applied to new circumstances? Or, have we shifted in important ways in regard to how we see our basic principles? Is patient autonomy simply a recent effort to express, perhaps no less clumsily, what we used to express by the Golden Rule? Or, is it something new in how we conceptualize the relationship of the nurse to the patient?

Notable constancies also can be found in the kinds of moral problems nurses face when entering the home in the context of health care services. There are issues of professional demeanor, relationships with other nurses and agencies, cooperation with physicians, relationships to family members, and the relationship to the patient. Many of these questions arise with much the same force and frequency as they did a century ago. Perhaps, this reflects important constancies in moral concerns and in the structure of daily life during the last century. Perhaps, too, it reflects the important role home care played at the turn of the century in the formation of nursing ethics.

The Primacy of Home Care Ethics

In 1900, home care, not hospital care, was the dominant form of nursing care, and hospital nursing did not become prominent until the advent of the scientific phase of nursing ethics in the 1940s. The coincidence of these two events is probably not incidental; for nurses to see hospitals as a better place than the home to express their ideals of caring, they may well have needed a more scientific and less personal outlook on ethics than the early nursing ethics literature provided. In 1900, nursing education took place primarily in hospitals; however, its concepts of professionalization were explicitly intended as preparation largely for work in the community as private duty nurse, visiting nurse, or public health nurse. As one might expect, the setting of home care placed an important mark on the early traditions of nursing ethics.

Indeed, early commentators on nursing ethics observed the important differences between home care and hospital care:

1. Assistance was not readily available and the nurse in need of help had to be resourceful.
2. The nurse had a single patient to be concerned with rather than many patients.
3. The nurse had more liberty in the home than in the hospital to organize the daily schedule (Robb, 1901, pp. 180–181).

All of these differences were, of course, only partially true at the turn of the century and now need serious modification: In cases of highly technical care in the home, the nurse may now be only one among many professionals who enters the home. Although the nurse may have a single patient in the home, she or he may now have several patients to see during a day's schedule, and a heavy schedule may restrict the nurse's options in planning the day.

In spite of these changes, a deep and important contrast still exists between hospital and home care nursing. When a nurse works in the hospital, he or she clearly works as part of an institution providing care. The various phases of care are divided into highly specialized roles. It can be argued that the institution as an organization is responsible for the care of the patient and that no particular person in the institution is responsible. Each professional is replaceable in a role just so long as those who fill the role practice professionally and competently. The ethics of the hospital is thus a formal ethics of role relations, legal responsibilities, and defined criteria. In the home, however, certainly at the turn of the century and now, if less distinctly, the professional provides care as an individual person. Not only did responsibility rest more distinctly on the individual practitioner, but also care was shaped and determined more strongly by the individual character of the practitioner. For this reason, and for others having to do with the roles of women one hundred years ago, ethics in home care was much more concerned at the turn of the century with the personality of the nurse.

Home Care and "Women's Work"

The history of nursing is closely tied to the history and status of women and women's work (Ashley, 1975). Since women's work has been traditionally rooted in the home, the role of the nurse in the home, even more than the nurse in the hospital, is closely related to women's work. To take just one dimension of this history, the "private duty" nurse at the turn of the century often lived in the home of the patient during the illness and recovery.* This had two immediate im-

* Similarly, nurses working in hospitals also lived in the hospital or a closely connected dormitory.

plications: first, the nurse was involved intimately in questions of housework, meals, and family life. Second, the nurse's private life was not very separate from her professional life, and so nursing ethics tended to comment on aspects of personal life as well as patient care duties.

Moreover, nurses in the home had to encounter directly one of the most difficult ethical binds facing workers. Traditionally and to a degree stereotypically, women have been the main proponents of ideals of a humane life, that is, ideals of service, self-sacrifice, community, caring, and concern for others. Men, as representatives of patriarchal traditions, also share in these ideals but have tended to stand, also somewhat stereotypically, for self-interest, power, violence, and aggression. This "yin" and "yang" of human duality has exploited women for their idealism.

Nursing in the home was initially closely related to housework:

> Job descriptions of the time appear to give major priority to scrubbing floors, dusting, keeping the stove stoked and the kerosene lamps trimmed and filled, controlling insects, washing clothes, making and rolling bandages, and other unskilled housekeeping tasks (Kelly, 1981, p. 45).

Housework is either unpaid work or the work of servants. Why, then, was a trained nurse to be paid more than a servant? Much of the work of nursing at the turn of the century was the work of establishing the value of the trained nurse—a higher-paid, educated nurse whose skills went well beyond a woman's "natural" (ie, unpaid) skills and justified pay, status, and professional respect. Throughout the century, nurses have worked in competition with less-trained practitioners who have done, or professed to do, similar women's work for less pay. Thus the private duty nurse was a more costly minority at the turn of the century in relation to the untrained, unpaid woman who worked as a "nightwatcher" sitting up with patients, sick care, housekeeping, and so forth. And, during the century nurses providing home care have worked in cooperation and competition with licensed practical nurses, wives, aunts, and other relatives, and similar poorly paid or unpaid workers.

This identification of nursing with these low-status jobs, tended to keep nursing from establishing itself independently of the patriarchal tradition in social relations and to keep private duty nurses from winning the rewards due them. Even though patriarchy has declined in the last century, and women everywhere are claiming the equality of status and rewards due them, the emphasis of the economy in the United States on self-interest, achievement, and consumerism still prevent work dedicated to service from receiving appropriate personal rewards. The problem in a nutshell, is this: how can nursing as a profession successfully stand for both just rewards for nurses and ideals of service in an economy founded on self-interest and exploitation as its basic modes of operation?

Sources of Information on Nursing Ethics in the Home

The discussion below relies primarily on two major sources: Isabel Hampton Robb's 1901 work on *Nursing Ethics: For Hospital and Private Use* and Charlotte Aikens' 1916 textbook *Studies in Ethics for Nurses*. Robb was a famous nursing leader and founder of important nursing schools, an innovator of curriculum, and an articulate proponent of the trained nurse. Aikens wrote a wide variety of textbooks after serving as a hospital and school director in a number of programs. Robb's book is beautifully written, and her ideas and words were imitated in many nursing articles of the time. Aikens' book expresses ideas very similar to Robb's. Aikens' book was intended as a textbook and apparently used widely, since it survived through at least five editions, the fifth in 1943. Aikens' book also has the advantage that it is richly supplied with cases on a wide range of themes. These cases are cited amply here for illustration. Since most of the cases were provided for students as exercises, it is sometimes difficult to say just how Aikens would analyze them. But it is usually possible to discern her views from the text of the book. Where she does not clarify a point, Robb's work often addresses the issue.

Although these two works form the central sources of this commentary, cases and text are included from a variety of other sources during the early years of nursing ethics.

RELATIONSHIP TO FAMILY

The relationship to the family (and other members of the household) is necessarily a complex one. On entering into family life, the nurse enters a microcosm of ethics that permits wide variability from one household to another. The nurse becomes another agent in an ongoing drama of several characters: What are the personal meanings to family members of the nurse's presence? How do the nurse's work and needs coordinate with the rest of the family? How does the family feel about the nurse? Who does patient care? How well? Who makes decisions about patient care? An early ethicist describes the situation as follows:

> You are brought into the heart of the family. Some of the members confide their domestic grievances to you. You will find a house divided against itself; 'for . . . there shall be five in one house divided

> three against two, and two against three. The mother shall be divided against the daughter, and the daughter against the other. The mother-in-law against her daughter-in-law, and the daughter-in-law against her mother-in-law.' Beware of taking sides. (Thompson, 1905, p. 164)

Aikens' cases on family life tend not so much to raise dilemmas for the nurse, but to rehearse parables in which the bottom line includes tact, propriety, and service.

Case 2–1. The Attentive Husband

> A nurse on an obstetrical case in a wealthy private home finds that the husband is very indifferent to wife and baby. The wife worries a good deal over his neglect. He is very profuse in his attentions to the nurse, insists on her always dining with him, and prolongs the meal hours as long as possible. The nurse knows how the wife feels about matters and is perplexed to know how to manage the situation. What suggestions can you offer her? (Aikens, 1916, p. 296)

This case involves a surprising number of themes: First, "meals are the cause of many disagreements that arise between nurse and family" (Aikens, 1916, p. 276), and nurses should be ready to accommodate family needs regarding their own meals. This permits the nurse a finesse: She can claim that she needs to be in the sickroom and must take her meals there. Second, the dangers of an inappropriate "tone and manner" (Aikens, 1916, p. 277) have already been amplified; for instance, a nurse should not call an adult male patient in his home by his first name. Lounsbery tackles the issue of intimacy unusually directly for the time:

> Never get into bed with your patient. . . . Never kiss the patient or allow yourself to show any demonstrative affection, unless you are very sure it will be welcome, and be careful even then. (Lounsbery, 1912, pp. 49, 57)

The dangers of conflict are especially great when "the woman who is the head of the home" becomes the patient (Aikens, 1916, p. 276). The ultimate failure for the nurse is being "sent away" and replaced by an untrained nurse, and so the case is something of a dilemma: The nurse could as easily be sent away by the husband as by the patient, especially since he is the patriarchal figure. I believe that it is clear in Aikens' writing that a bearing inspiring confidence and service to the patient are key, so that the nurse should risk offending the husband to reduce jealousy in the household.

Jealousy in relationship to the woman of the house is an important psychic theme, since the woman of the house is powerless when ill, and the nurse is being paid to do her work. To indicate the durability of the problem, Bermosk and Corsini in their 1973 collection present an incident in which they describe the feelings of failure on the part of a sick child's mother because a nurse has been called in to assist (Bermosk & Corsini, 1973).

Reputation

Let us turn to a somewhat different case involving children.

Case 2–2. Small Lies

> As soon as the mother has gone, the nurse telephones to the city and invites two friends to spend the day with her. She bribes the little girl not to tell her mother. Comment on the nurse's actions in this case. Would they tend to increase the confidence and respect accorded to trained nurses in that town? (Aikens, 1916, p. 296)

Like the first case, this case is not a dilemma. The nursing student was expected to know the answer to the question, and the resolution of the problem is in terms of "confidence and respect accorded to trained nurses" and not in terms of a more abstract duty of honesty. Not only was the reputation of the two nurses at stake, but the reputation of trained nurses in general was also. In a passage warning nurses "never to take a single glass of wine," Robb emphasized the crucial importance of reputation in the work of private nurses:

> The trained nurse occupies a position in which she is subjected to constant watching and criticism, and I know of no class of men or women who are expected to walk more circumspectly or more worthy of their vocation. (Robb, 1901, p. 238)

The case is poignant in a way, because nurses living in patients' homes had few opportunities for recreation. Robb recommended that recreation be arranged away from the home and that alternate care for the patient be arranged with the family for a friend or family member to take her place (Robb, 1901, p. 243). This nurse's activities failed on both counts.*

---

* This writer notes that she was dealing with two children. Her great mistake was not to bribe both of them.

The Family After the Patient Dies

Case 2–3. The Funeral

A patient, an elderly man, dies. The body is to be shipped out of the city for burial. The only daughter of the deceased is to accompany the body, leaving the widow, an elderly woman, alone. The daughter asks the nurse to stay with her mother till she returns from the funeral. There is nothing for the nurse to do but ordinary household duties and to serve as companion for the old lady. Should the nurse stay? (Aikens, 1916, p. 299)

Questions regarding the duty of private nurses to deceased patients and their families continued to arise during the century. This case turns on questions of the nature of the nursing service in the home. First, since the nurse was doing "sick" care, activities in cleaning up the room after a death, preparing the body, and so forth, fall outside the narrow concept of sick care. Yet, there are many things that need to be done in relationship to a death that a nurse could do.

The nurse's duty to the remaining family is also unclear, and this unclarity is a common one in health care. Was the nurse caring for just the patient, or the patient and the family? Nursing ethics permitted a broad interpretation of what could be done for the patient, but could these broad tasks be extended to performing household duties for the family members? The problem is difficult because Robb was very clear that the nurse in the home must maintain a discreet relationship with the family: "She should never fail to preserve the little invisible line of reserve" (Robb, 1901, p. 242). The nurse is there for the patient. This means that the nurse should be unobtrusive, but at the same time she should manage the family's relationship to the patient. Once her job is done, she should not maintain a relationship with the family or patient (except perhaps a brief courtesy call) and certainly should not stay on in the household until another case arises. The situation calls for "a businesslike promptness in coming and going" (Robb, 1901, p. 244). Since Robb has made this claim so strong, the nurse needs some justification to remain with the family. Indeed, if the contract was with the male head of household (now deceased), the nurse may have found that staying on involved reduced wages for the less valuable activities of keeping relatives company.

The ethical question arose long before professionals created concepts of family nursing, family practice, family health, family dynamics, and certainly before psychological study of stages of grieving, normal grief, grief therapy, etc. The advent of more technical approaches to grief and family relations permit interpreting such activities as professional work and make the transition less difficult. In spite of these developments toward professionalizing emotional experience, the role of nurses, whether in the hospital or in the home, in social arrangements and referrals is still often unclear.

The Character of the Nurse

Case 2–4. The Stern Nurse

A well-to-do family (not rich) living in an apartment house had occasion to call a nurse for the mother of the lady of the house, an old lady in the eighties, who was slowly dying of some form of cancer—no external wounds. The man of the house was obliged to take business trips out of the city which often kept him away for weeks. He thought a trained nurse would be a pleasant companion for his wife. The nursing duties were light, but he did not care to have his wife left alone. No maid was kept. The nurse came, a stern, unbending creature who literally took possession of the sickroom and, from the moment she entered, gave the lady of the house to understand that she would tolerate no trespassing on her domain. Neither did she intend to offer to do anything outside the actual care of the patient. . . . The daughter prepared more elaborate meals for herself and the nurse than she would have done when she was alone, washed the dishes and waited on the nurse instead of on her mother. . . . At the end of two weeks the husband returned, and finding that his wife was working harder than before the nurse came and the mother missed her daughter so sorely, dispensed with the nurse's services. A few days later they secured an untrained woman who fitted into the household as if she belonged there, assisted the daughter with the nursing and with any other duty that had to be done, and remained with the family till the patient died. What were the chief reasons for the failure of the trained nurse in this case? (Aikens, 1916, pp. 299–300)

A number of points are noteworthy here. First, we again see the importance of the untrained nurse as a threatening figure (a boogeyperson) who enforces compliance. Second, the nurse's major fault was her personality, not her professional competence. She was a "stern unbending creature"; she was neither unprincipled nor irresponsible; indeed, she was serious in adherence to the duties of patient care. Third, she did not permit "trespassing on her domain," when she should have allowed family members access to the patient. Nurses were expected to control the access of the family to the patient and to supervise family care of the patient, but this was to be done tactfully and unobtrusively:

> . . . she has to select the most competent members of the family as her assistant, to work under her instructions, or to relieve her when off duty for her necessary rest or recreation. . . . Where the family are inclined to interfere with her orders for her patient, it will be best for her to ask the doctor to write down the necessary instructions, or to insist upon them to the friends. (Robb, 1901, pp. 240–41)

Fourth, the daughter was required to labor on behalf of the nurse to meet the nurse's needs. Aikens warned:

> Many nurses seem to feel that the family that is employing them owes them exactly the same attention and deference that would be shown to a guest. (p. 274)

Robb also warned nurses against developing habits of self-indulgence lest "her increased demands and lessened capacity finally render her undesirable to physicians and to all classes of patients" (Robb, 1901, p. 238). As we finish with this set of cases, the reference in Aiken above to the status of "guest" raises one of the key problems in defining the ethics of home care: What is the status in the home and family of the nurse? Is she a guest, a friend, a family member, a visitor, a spy, a servant, or other? In the early part of the century, we find the beginnings of the concept of the professional in the home, a role that is continuing to be redefined. In the words of Robb:

> In private families, outside the sickroom, it was hard to know what to do with her. She was neither for the kitchen nor for the drawing-room—neither fish, flesh nor fowl—and she was often placed in positions that required from her not only tact but a large amount of forbearance. (p. 32)

PROFESSIONALISM

Most striking in the history of professionalism in nursing is that nursing has continued to be described as "just emerging" as a profession throughout the last century. During this century, nurses increasingly enhanced their basic education and qualifications, strengthened their professional organizations, increased their autonomy in the workplace and their personal control over their private time, enhanced their status, articulated the ethics and purpose of their professional commitment, and improved their job security, rewards, and career opportunities. At the same time, the definition of "profession" continued to shift toward more restrictive criteria, and older, higher-status, and male-dominated professions continued to outpace nursing in many of these areas of professional gain. Thus, it has been possible for nurses and others to describe themselves as professionals one hundred years ago, and yet the profession can still be patronized as a "semi-profession" today (Moore, 1988).

The professionalization of nursing during the last century necessarily involved progress in ethics as it defined the profession of nursing. Early nurses therefore encountered a variety of questions having to do with relationship to other professions, to other nurses, to uniforms, fees, tips, competition, agencies, and confidentiality, to list a few of the major professional issues.

Relationship to Servants

If the unpaid female family member was one important model from which to distinguish nurses, the paid household servant was another. The confusion was inevitable. Nursing as a profession is partly an outgrowth of the work of nursemaids, nighwatchers, nursery maids, and other household servants (Reverby, 1987). Although household workers were and are dignified persons who do worthy work, this work has not normally received the rewards it should. A servant is extremely dependent on his or her employer, and to be a servant is to suffer "long hours, poor pay, and miserable conditions" (Martin & Segrave, 1985 p. *v*). In addition to defining a professional concept of service to patients, nurses were also trying to define more adequate and fair rewards for themselves. The model of servant was thus a threat to rewards for nurses. It was indeed a double hazard because nursery maids and the like were low-status servants as compared to higher-status, usually male, servants such as butlers and chauffeurs (Huggett, 1977). We thus find cases involving the nurse's relationship to the servants.

Case 2–5. The Maid Has the Grippe

> A nurse is called to care for two elderly ladies who are ill with bronchitis. The maid, the only other member of the household, develops grippe and goes to her sister's. Outline the nurse's duties under such circumstances. (Aikens, 1916, p. 294)

It was Aikens' position in 1916 that the distinction between nurse and domestic servant was already sufficiently established and that any confusion between the two was already 50 years out of date, with the result that a nurse who did occasional domestic labor was still clearly identifiable as a nurse in 1916. However, private duty nurses continued to fear this confusion, and so there is reason to suspect that the confusion still persisted. Aikens held that, instead of standing on dignity, the nurse was to respond to the Nightingale model and to "labor for the good of the sick to the utmost of her power." The basic rule, in Aikens' view, was,

> There is nothing which needs to be done for the comfort of any patient which it is beneath my dignity to do. (p. 272)

Indeed, Aikens attempted to cast contempt on the whole issue, even though it continued to persist in the literature into the 1960s.*

Case 2–6. Washing Diapers

A young graduate on her first obstetrical case was asked by the young mother if she would wash out the baby's fine woolen shirts in the bathroom, and stretch them carefully while drying. . . . The young nurse was not sure whether this duty came in her province or not, but she finally decided to do it, and then try to find out what the custom of other nurses was in regard to such matters. The incident assumed an importance in her mind out of all proportion to the matter involved, which was a simple act of kindness. Two nurses whom she consulted said she should not have done it, that, she was "lowering the standards of the profession," a third one thought she did right, said she would have done the same thing. To settle the disputed question, the young nurse finally wrote to the office of a nursing magazine for an opinion as to whether she did right or wrong to wash out those little shirts. The whole question was so unimportant as to seem unworthy of any sincere group of women, who desired to be treated as professional people. (Aikens, 1916, p. 271)

Robb also seemed to believe that the nurses' higher status was well established at the turn of the century:

> The trained nurse, then, is no longer to be regarded as a better trained, more useful, higher class servant, but as one who has knowledge and is worthy of respect, consideration and due recompense—in a certain degree a member of a profession. (Robb, 1901, p. 37)

---

* Interestingly, the phrases "But a half century has wrought marked social changes, . . . [and] [t]he social status of the nurse has been established" (Aikens, 1916, p. 272) recur unchanged in the fifth edition of the text 26 years later. Did time stand still?

Secure in this position, she also clearly included the daily care of the patient's room among distinctively nursing duties. Besides being ethical, it was more efficient:

> The building of a grate-fire for instance, if done intelligently, is a matter of a few minutes to the nurse, and the quiet of the sickroom is not invaded, whereas the importation of an ignorant servant from the kitchen, with the necessary appliances, may require a great deal more effort and time, as well as much disturbance, to the patient, nurse and family. (Robb, 1901, p. 223)

Robb was partly concerned with encouraging nurses to care for their own needs and to avoid burdening family and serving staff, partly with the same openness to patients' needs that Aikens encouraged:

> . . . the performance of any manner of service that can in any way be of benefit or relief to her patient, or that will save life; nor should she waste her time in debating every case whether this or that particular service comes under the head of nursing duties, or should be relegated to the servants. (Robb, 1901, p. 228)

This issue persisted into the 1960s at least. The *American Journal of Nursing* "Open Forum" responded to the same question in 1934.

Case 2–7. Cleaning the Floor

> How much of the cleaning of a patient's room is expected of a private duty nurse, that is, sweeping of floors, dusting, et cetera? If the patient is on a regular diet is the nurse expected to prepare the same?

The editor responded that cases had to be considered individually, but the bottom line was that if it were helpful to the patient and there was no one else to do it, the editor hoped, "we would doff our uniform and get on with the scrubbing."

Spalding, writing in the post-1939 "scientific" period of nursing ethics, answered the question in exactly the same way:

> The question frequently comes up as to whether or not the nurse should perform certain acts which, strictly speaking, are not those of nursing. . . . While it is true that, as a nurse, you would not be expected to provide purely a maid service there are certainly some services which a patient may expect from you. . . . A good principle to follow is to do whatever is needed for the patient's physical, mental and spiritual comfort. (Spalding, 1939, p. 379)

In spite of vast changes in title and content of the Spalding work from the 1939 first edition to the 1970 eighth edition, this paragraph persisted unchanged through the 1965 seventh edition until it was completely dropped in the eighth.

Working Hours

Returning to the problem in Case 2–5, the basic principle was being put under pressure. It is one thing for the nurse to do occasional incidental duties; what if a full-time maid is needed? The concern in this case shifted from the definition of the role to the level of labor required of the nurse. In the story, she already had two patients. Are there limits to the work load of a nurse?

This is a difficult question to answer. The early writers on ethics encouraged nurses to maintain their own health, to rest, to reduce stress, to exercise, to eat properly, to sleep well, to take regular vacations, and not to nurse relatives during vacations. Despite this, there was little discussion during the early years of nursing ethics regarding working hours, a right to rest, or limits on the work week. Instead, nurses were expected not to exercise control of their own hours, with disastrous consequences for nurses.

The private duty nurse was apparently usually on duty twenty-four hours a day for the duration of a case. Long hours were by far the main reason nurses were planning to leave private duty, according to the Burgess survey (Burgess, 1926). Over half of private duty cases in the home were for twenty-four-hour duty, the balance for twelve-hour day or night shifts (Burgess, 1928, p. 302). These shifts seldom included proper rest:

> 12 hour day duty is usually thought of as including two hours of rest, although nurses testify that in practice they are frequently unable to secure any such free period. Twenty-four-hour duty in theory includes four hours of rest and at least a few hours of sleep at night. Here, again, however, nurses report that in many cases they are unable to get either free time in the day or an adequate amount of sleeping time at night. (Burgess, 1928, p. 302)

Private duty nurses addressing the issue of hours described them as "ghastly," "hideous," "a slave's life," and "inhuman." Nurses were "wrecked" by hard cases and "bored" by easy ones. They got little sleep, suffered health problems, went home exhausted and worn out, were lonely and unable to socialize, were unable to plan their time, lacked sunshine and recreation, could not attend church or social meetings, lacked reading and exposure to culture, and in general lacked "anything a human being ought to have in this world" (Burgess, 1928, pp. 322–329).

At the time of Burgess' study, the recently common concept of going from home to home and spending a few hours with each patient was confined to public health and visiting nursing. For a patient to receive a few hours of care from several nurses, which is now the agency norm, was a new idea that interested nurses but was little practiced and was termed "hourly" and "group" nursing (Burgess, 1928).

The model of the hospital nurse at this time offered the private duty nurse little comfort and set few limits on working hours. Nursing students functioning as apprentices were expected to work nine to thirteen hours a day, six days a week, for low "training" wages and then to attend classes as well. A passage in Robb's work is revealing.

Case 2–8. The Overly Conscientious Nurse

> Thus, it not infrequently occurs that a head-nurse directs a probationer to leave the ward at a certain hour; the probationer, however, finding there is still much work to be done, probably out of mistaken kindness, or from a desire to help, takes it upon herself to remain beyond her time, until she is finally ordered off with a gentle reproof or the request to do only what she is told. (Robb, 1901, p. 58)

This was an opportunity for Robb to speak of a nurse's entitlement to rest and time off; instead, she reproved the probationer (ie, beginning student) for failing to maintain "implicit obedience and a habit of strictly minding one's own affairs." Although significant nursing leaders, such as Mary Adelaide Nutting, supported limitations on hours, the early writers on ethics, as do many current writers on the subject, focused on the duties of nurses and not on their rights.

Most of the reforms of working hours came from outside of nursing. Trade unions were involved in negotiations and legislation limiting the work week, and during the second decade of this century, a California law limiting the work week was applied to hospital nurses and apprentices. Opposition from hospitals led to a Supreme Court case concerning the inclusion of nursing apprentices in the legislation. Many nurses opposed the limits on working hours because they resented being identified with trade unionists, and in the words of one nursing leader, hoped to resolve the issue in "a more dignified manner" (Ashley, 1976). Although the move to control hours in the hospital was successful, the limitations were not applied to private duty nursing in homes. Thus the concept of professionalism was working here against the welfare of individual nurses rather than improving their status. These early definitions of professionalism by nursing ethicists thus permitted exploitation of nurses through long hours and an indefinite commitment to manual labor. Robb summed up this function of ethics:

> But there is another side to nursing—the ethical—without which all the work accomplished would be dead and spiritless, and which is the antidote for a too pronounced professional attitude. From this standpoint the nurse's work is a ministry; it should represent a consecrated service, performed in the spirit of Christ, who made himself of no account but went about doing good. (Robb, 1901, pp. 37–38)

Cooperation Among Nurses and Equitable Access to Care

A key feature of professionalism involves its definition of the relationship of nurses to each other in their work. Cooperation and competition among agencies, registries, schools, and individual nurses were thus common topics for ethical concern in nursing's early years. Different types of home care were a common source of controversy.

Case 2–9. The Visiting Nurse

A visiting nurse is employed by a committee of ladies for service in a town of 3500. Two graduate nurses whose homes are in or near the town are practicing there and are busy, a considerable part of their work being maternity nursing. . . . [The committee is] to pay her $65* a month, but she is supposed to earn most of it. The committee announces through the press that they are providing a nurse for the poor. They announce to the visiting nurse that they expect her to secure as much work as she possibly can from people who are able to pay, and that the continuance of her service there depends on how much she herself can earn toward her own salary. Through their clubs and churches and friends the committee advertises the benefits of their visiting nurse, and prospective mothers are urged to secure her for service at birth and for as many hours daily thereafter as they need. The visiting work, through the advertising given and the activity of the committee, enjoys a 'boom'; the work of the two private nurses dwindles. They go to the visiting nurse and complain that she is cutting rates, spending whole days at cases, and taking away their work. She explains that she has to do this work in order to keep her position, and that the committee fixes her rates. What should the visiting nurse do and what should the private nurses do under such circumstances? (Aikens, 1916, p. 292)

* The $65 per month figure became $150 per month in the 1943 edition.

In 1916, there were no government-supported programs like Medicare and Medicaid providing money to pay for the care of needy persons and families; employer-supported health insurance programs were also at a bare minimum. The pressure on nurses to do charitable work was thus great. In her text, Aikens noted the great need for obstetrical services in the home. She also stressed that nurses should provide some free care as part of their professional activities:

> It should be made a matter of principle every year for a nurse to render a certain amount of service for which she never expects to be paid—. . . the principle that every nurse in common with every other right-minded individual owes every year some measure of free service to humanity cannot be easily reasoned away. (Aikens, 1916, p. 253)

How much care, whether a nurse should ever work below contract, etc., Aikens regarded as "vexed questions" beyond the scope of her text.* The private nurses in the case above had thus missed an opportunity to be doing charity work in this town, particularly, obstetrical work. She would also, with Robb, urge the nurses to deal with their conflict respectfully:

> Their professional relations should be marked by mutual courtesy, respect and good-fellowship; and no personal feelings should ever be permitted to interfere with their work. (Robb, 1901, p. 259)

The only really well established competition-reducing principle was expressed by Robb and was referred to in a number of cases—the first-come, first-serve rule:

> When two or more nurses are engaged to take care of a patient in a private family, it is the rule that the one who arrives first should take charge of the case, the second acting as her assistant. (Robb, 1901, p. 260)

Similarly, since obtaining a nurse might take several calls, a second nurse could easily arrive to a case where another had already responded. The first to arrive, of course, got the case. Unfortunately, this rule was not useful in the above case, and resolution of it needed strong cooperation among nurses, probably with the aid of a professional or labor organization.

This case has relevance for ethics in home care today, since agencies experience competition among public and private services, among

---

* This remark is strange, because Aikens regarded very little as beyond the scope of her text.

subsidized and unsubsidized services, and among agencies facing different costs of doing business.

Fees for Nursing Services

Price competition was more difficult, however. It was a practice of some schools to run home care services with their students as workers, and their graduates in practice objected strongly. Private duty nurses were also in steady competition with untrained nurses and needed to justify their higher fees. Although a few wealthy families could pay handsomely for nursing care, middle-class and poor families had to stretch budgets to obtain nursing care, and the ever-sympathetic nurse aspired to avoid being a financial burden on her clients.

In Case 2–8, the new nursing service was presented as a charitable enterprise, but it was also a way for higher-class consumers to combine to obtain cheaper services for those of their own class. The bulk of the nurse's work was to be regular private duty work for pay at a cut rate to recover her salary. There is no way the nurse could then also provide care for the poor without working overtime at a reduced rate. The new nurse was thus being exploited, and it would be important for the private duty nurses to point this out to her.

Issues such as these needed an active nursing association or labor organization able to assist the nurses in working together rather than against each other. Although 1916 was a period of extremely active labor organization against price competition among workers, we can find barely a breath of such concerns in the ethics texts.

One result of this generous outlook was that the salaries of nurses in general, and private duty nurses in particular, tended to lag behind those of other workers. By the mid 1920s, for instance, the private duty nurse tended to make less money and to save less than her hospital counterparts. On the average, she worked for pay 7 months a year, contributed a month's work in charity, and was idle the remaining 4 months of the year (Burgess, 1928, p. 310). She received on average $1,311 per year as compared to the hospital nurse, who made $2,079 per year (Burgess, 1928, p. 305).

Robb articulated the classical professional position toward the relationship between service and financial reward:

> It is clearly not only allowable but praiseworthy that a nurse should receive as compensation for her work not only a present livelihood for herself, and something additional to bestow on others, but that she should also be able to make provision for her old age, when she would otherwise have to depend on the labor of others. Her nursing need not necessarily suffer because she receives pay for it. But . . . if the pecuniary considerations are in her mind of primary importance, then all the beauty of the life is gone. (Robb, 1901, p. 203)

She recommended not being too critical of the beginning nurse in whom "the commercial instinct seemed to be unpleasantly prominent," and she was clear that the work called for "no niggardly compensation." She suggested a base pay of $3.00 per day* and a sliding scale of reductions for families unable to pay that much. For families able to pay, she "is justified in asking for the maximum rate" and:

> it is only just and wise that she should receive her due, and that she not allow those who are well able to pay for her services to take up her time without proper recompense, and thus prevent her from helping the poor and needy in their turn. (Robb, 1901, p. 207)

Three important points are of interest here. First, we note in the last line, the expectation that nurses would charge the rich in order to serve the poor. This expresses a long-established custom of using "cost-shifting" to increase equity in access to health care. This ethical commitment was apparently not extremely successful, since only about 1 percent of the poor were able to obtain private duty nurses as compared to about 12 percent of those in higher income levels (Fowler, 1984, p. 183). Despite the justice of the custom, it has come under attack recently, primarily by insurance companies, with negative effects on the ability of the health care system to respond to the poor.

Second, Robb articulates the important principle of justice in health policy that the quality of care not be linked to the ability of the patient to pay:

> But no matter what is the rate of remuneration agreed upon, let the nurse see to it that her services are suited to the exigencies of the disease and are not regulated by the worldly means of the sufferer. (Robb, 1901, p. 206)

Third, Robb expresses a key ideal of professionalism: Place service before personal income. Indeed, her claims for the income of nurses is quite modest; it includes nothing for prestige, for education, or for status in relationship to other workers. At least she shows respect for personal rewards for nurses and defines a concept of salary above that needed for survival.

For the most part, the ethics literature tends to place the private duty nurse in a passive position in regard to salary. Aikens, for instance, articulated no principle of financial reward for nurses and focused instead on methods of living within a limited income—savings, budgeting, and personal economy. Similarly, a 1931 *American*

* I presume she is referring to a twenty-four-hour day.

Journal of Nursing column received a question from a public health nurse as to what she should do when a family had enough money to pay the doctor, but not enough to pay the nurse. The editor responded that the problem was not one for the individual nurse but is a problem for the agency to resolve, which, the column recommended, should have a medical advisory board (*American Journal of Nursing*, 1931). This passive approach to income and instruction on living within limits persisted in the Spalding 1939 text, in spite of its broader look at nursing status, organization, and income.

The questions that came up in ethics settings about salary more often cover the details of payment: Can a nurse accept gifts or tips? Who should pay for travel costs, especially if the family refuses the nurse on arrival? Aikens, not surprisingly, warns against accepting money tips for extra services, and although less strict about accepting small nonmonetary gifts, she warns against soliciting them (Aikens, 1916, pp. 74–75).

Relations with Physicians

This is a chapter of shame in the history of home care ethics. In relationship to the physician, the nurse was sold into slavery by nursing's own leaders. In so doing, the nursing profession, with the ample support of physicians and hospitals, shares responsibility for carrying the tradition of patriarchal control in health care well into the late Twentieth Century.

At the turn of the century, private duty nurses worked closely with physicians in the home as well as in the hospital, since the home visit was a common practice of physicians. Because the Flexner report did not come out until 1910, most nurses in the home worked primarily with physicians trained in non-Flexnerian medical schools. These physicians were highly variable in their competence, and a substantial number were wholly unprepared scientifically. Private duty nurses must therefore have witnessed many instances of incompetent medical care. Indeed, the growth of nursing and its witnessing of poor quality of care may have been an important force toward placing medical training on a more scientific basis, but if so, this force was imposed very, very quietly (Fowler, 1984, p. 178).

The early nursing ethics literature included ample numbers of cases concerning the competence of the physician. However, it gave little or no guidance on how to cope with poor-quality medical care, and instead, placed the nurse in a virtually impossible bind of strong conflicting loyalties to patient and to physician. One source of this difficulty is that the early ethics literature said very little about the nurse's responsibility for her own competence. One cannot find the language of "excellence" in skills or care, "quality of care," or "competence." Instead, the notion of high character, dedication, and moral integrity mostly substituted conceptually for the concept of competence. For instance, Robb defined professionalism primarily in terms of "vocation" or "calling." Her reference to "a higher skill and an employment needing an education more thorough than that required in some other vocations in life" (Robb, 1901, p. 33) is of course implicit in all she said, but Robb interpreted the nurse's response to her responsibility for competence mainly in terms of her obedience, her ability to follow instructions, and her personal integrity rather than in extensive attention to self-correction, development of skills, and establishing standards of quality. Gradually, this ethical approach to competence was set aside in favor of a more technical approach. For instance, Aikens left "profession" undefined in her 1916 work, but by her fifth edition, in 1943, she characterized the concept primarily in terms of skills and training:

> A profession may be defined as an occupation requiring a background of education and culture, combined with special skills, and calling for discipline and standards suitable to an important vocation. (p. 28)

Spalding (1939, p. 38) gave a very similar definition. This increasing focus on the technical in professionalism continued into the 1990s. The 1985 American Nurses' Association Code for Nurses placed substantial emphasis on nursing competence and expected educational qualifications of the nurse continue to increase (American Nurses' Association, 1985).

The real issue, however, is one of responsibility for quality, and the early nurse was placed in an impossible bind. First, Robb modeled responsibility for quality in the home on nursing responsibility in the hospital. In distinguishing the role of the nurse from the physician, Robb claimed that,

> . . . during long months of training in the hospital she [the nurse] has not only had careful instruction on these points, but has also had opportunities every day of appreciating the necessary distinctions and how this recognition should influence her own conduct. (Robb, 1901, p. 249)

The key virtue for nurses in the hospital was obedience:

> Above all, let her remember to do what she is told to do, and no more; the sooner she learns this lesson, the easier her work will be for her, and the less likely will she be to fall under severe criticism. Implicit, unquestioning obedience is one of the first lessons a probationer must learn, for this is a quality that will be expected from her in her professional capacity for all future time. (Robb, 1901, p. 57)

Robb carried this obligation of obedience in the hospital over to home care in relationship to the physician:

> . . . the physician is primarily and ultimately responsible for the life and health of the patient, and that it necessarily follows that the direction of the treatment belongs to him; and secondly, that the nurse, acting as his assistant, is bound to carry out this treatment loyally and faithfully without modifying it or changing it in any way. (Robb, 1901, p. 250)

Robb's advice was incredibly strong in this direction:

> Granted, even, that the physician in a given case may not be skillful—and on this point, I would insist again, the nurse is not always competent to judge—the responsibility for his engagement lies with the patient or his friends, and information as to his incompetency should never come from the nurse. (Robb, 1901, p. 253)

A significant irony in these claims is that the home care nurse was held personally responsible for any poor care she might provide and that neither physician nor agency was likely to be held responsible for damage done by her. Thus the legal risks in obeying incompetent orders fell on the nurse. The nurse was in a classical position of responsibility without authority. One argument used by hospitals to waive responsibility for the nurse's actions was that the nurse was a professional (Goodhart, 1938, p. 553). The private duty nurse was even more likely to be seen as an independent contractor, and registries tended to be held legally responsible only for listing qualified nurses and not for the actions of those nurses.

The legal and ethical traditions thus placed the nurse in a position of dependency on the male-dominated profession of medicine. This situation did not go unprotested by early nurses such as Lavinia Dock and Isabel Stewart but the writers on ethics provided little aid or comfort for nurses. Robb reminded private duty nurses that they were dependent on physicians for calls and so,

> . . . a nurse's chance for future work can often be affected disastrously, if a doctor has reason to suspect her disloyalty or if she appears to be overstepping what he considers to be her professional province. It is a rather one-sided loyalty that the physician demands. He often sees no reason why he should be loyal to the nurse, while he is quick to condemn her for apparent disloyalty to him. (Robb, 1916, p. 278)

Despite this tradition of dependency, the question of quality of care had to be dealt with. Aikens faced the issue more squarely than

Robb and, to her credit, raised the key question. After quoting a physician who equated loyalty to physician with loyalty to patient, she asked: "Does loyalty to the physician and faithfulness to the patient always mean one and the same thing?" Without directly responding to the question with a resounding "No," she raised cases in which it was patent that the two are not identical.

Case 2–10. Abdominal Trouble

> A nurse is called to care for a patient who appears to be suffering from some abdominal trouble. The patient is of a nervous type and has been operated on for abdominal trouble less than two years previously. The doctor suggests another operation.* The patient protests against it and the doctor demands that a consultant be called. He [ie, the doctor] is given permission to choose his own consultant and they exactly agree as to diagnosis and treatment. The husband of the patient is far from satisfied that an operation is needed. The nurse is not supposed to diagnose, but she can hardly help forming an opinion as to whether the operation is as urgently needed as the doctor suggests. The patient and husband both look to her for some suggestion. What should she do? (Aikens, 1916, pp. 278–279)

Admittedly, Aikens believed that the nurse should not be open in disagreements with physicians. She described a case in which a physician prescribed a nutrient enema for a gastric ulcer to be preceded by a soap-and-water injection. The nurse sent a note to the physician, in which she diagnosed anemia and a fecal impaction. She recommended poultices of "hot linseed with a little turpentine" and doses of castor oil. Aikens asked nursing students to state reasons for disapproving of the note and to reflect on the lack of virtues in the nurse (Aikens, 1916, pp. 289–290). Clearly, the nurse had overstepped the scope of her practice. The ethical commitment to silence continued well into the century. For instance, Spalding stated what had been held for the previous half-century:

> But she would not make a formal diagnosis or prescribe medical treatment other than might be considered safe in home or in emergency treatment (Spalding, 1939, p. 337).

---

* Remember that we are talking about early years of surgical practice when anesthesia and asepsis were of poor quality.

The following case combined questions about coping with medical incompetence with questions of cooperation in an "unethical" procedure.

Case 2–11. An Abortion

A nurse is called to nurse a case of septicemia following abortion. The patient, a young married woman, is very ill, and confesses to the nurse that she wished she had never had the abortion performed. It is evident that the doctor in charge of the case is the one who secured the abortion, though the patient does not plainly say so. The doctor appears to be attentive to the case, but thoroughly incompetent. The nurse feels that under different management the patient might have a chance to recover. What is her duty in the matter? (Aikens, 1916, p. 279)

On arrival at the case, the nurse had an option of refusing the case because an abortion was involved, and she need not have worked with the physician again. However, the patient needed her help and the nurse was not to criticize the physician. The nurse's only remaining recourse, therefore, was to hint to the patient that another physician might be called to consult.

Case 2–12. Dirty Hands

A visiting nurse is engaged by a family to assist at a birth and to visit the patient afterward. The doctor's manner when she arrives shows very plainly that he does not wish the nurse to assist him in any way. She offers to prepare a disinfectant solution for his hands, asks whether he wishes anything sterilized, etc. He gruffly declines any such suggestions and does not even wash his hands before making an examination to determine progress of labor. What should the nurse do in such a case during the labor? If a septic condition follows the birth in such a case, and the nurse knows the doctor is careless or incompetent, what are her duties in the matter? (Aikens, 1916, pp. 291–292)

Aikens and other ethics writers offered many other such cases, which we need not detail here. They involved nurses who would have liked to refer patients to physicians of better quality, who wanted to make suggestions to physicians, who needed to cope with incompetent physicians, and who considered talking with patients and families about the physician. One nurse was asked by the family of a patient to attend a postmortem to keep an eye on the physicians.

An *American Journal of Nursing* case raised the question of staying on a case when a physician is discharged (*American Journal of Nursing*, 1927). This appears to have been a delicate issue. The nurse had to first check with the physician to make sure that he did not want her to leave the case as soon as she was not needed. Then, if she stayed on, she needed to check with the incoming physician to see if he wanted her to remain on the case. Edgell raised a somewhat different kind of conflict in 1929.

Case 2–13. Unjustified Suffering

> . . . a nurse [is] ordered by a doctor to take tests on a patient at prescribed intervals. The patient is dying, he has suffered greatly and is now lying in a semiconscious condition; in order to take the prescribed test it will be necessary to stimulate the patient and bring him back again to a consciousness of pain. What ought the nurse to do? She does not know the purpose of the test and cannot judge the importance or unimportance of a record from this particular patient. (Edgell, 1929, p. 100)

Here, the nurse suspected that an ethical problem was present, and although she understood that a good reason for the test was possible, she felt uncomfortable in causing the patient suffering without having a better understanding herself of the need for the test. Since most early writers on nursing ethics referred to the problem of conflicts with physicians regarding the quality of care, we must conclude that the issue came up frequently (Dietz, 1939; Parsons, 1916). And, in spite of strong statements of loyalty to physicians, nurses were not left without recourse by early ethicists. Although restricted from sharing their concern with patients, nurses had several options. They could and should refuse to work with a physician they regarded as incompetent (Robb, 1901, p. 251) and certainly should refuse to work with irregular, unlicensed practitioners; they could and should speak with the physician regarding their reservations (Parsons, 1916, p. 58); they could recommend a consultation if questioned persistently by the family (Robb, 1901, p. 252); and in difficult cases, they could confer with the head of their registry or the director of their school (Spalding, 1939, p. 382). Even so, private duty nurses' options were very restricted. Spalding well characterizes the spirit of the situation:

> . . . if you should become convinced of inefficiency or malpractice on the part of a physician. No one formula can serve on all occasions, but in any event it is obvious that considerable tact and judgment must be employed. No nurse should openly defame or criticize a physician. . . . In a private family, of course, this problem becomes even more difficult. You cannot just leave the patient because the physician in charge is not worthy of his profession. Here you must remember your responsibility to the patient, who, in the hands of a quack or an unethical practitioner, needs your service more than ever. . . . You cannot sit idly by when you are convinced of malpractice, and so you must do all in your power, tactfully, of course, to bring about a consultation. One way of arranging this might be to ask a priest or minister to suggest it. (Spalding, 1939, p. 382)

The professional issue of quality of care was not the only one to concern early nursing ethicists. Another area of nurse–physician relationships focused on personal relations between nurses and physicians. The patriarchal tradition traded to some degree on a failure to distinguish between the personal and the professional authority of the physician. For the protection of the nurse, the nursing ethicists recommend great caution and propriety in this realm. Aikens reported a rule for nurses in training that they not visit doctors in their offices nor consult them without consulting the principal of the school first. This rule was intended in part to prevent the development of personal relationships. For instance,

> . . . one of the visiting doctors was in the habit of making visits after ten o'clock at night, and of spending an hour or more in 'visiting' with the senior night nurse who was serving as night supervisor. After this nurse came off night duty, she paid frequent evening calls to this same physician in his office. When asked the reason for these visits, she stated that the doctor was treating her for headache and throat trouble. (Aikens, 1916, p. 149)

Inevitably, such problems also turned up for private duty nurses.

Case 2–14. The Attentive Physician

A doctor (married) who frequently employs a nurse for private duty is inclined to be familiar in his manner. He visits the patient, presumably, but spends twice as much time with the nurse as with the patient. The nurse is afraid the patient will think she is to blame for the doctor spending most of the time spent in the call with her. She does not wish to offend the doctor because he sends her many calls, but she is determined that her name shall not be connected with this doctor's as a topic for neighborhood gossip. How shall she manage this problem? (Aikens, 1916, p. 302)

Aikens also told of a problem with a pharmacist who substituted inferior drugs for those ordered. He sent bottles of perfume to the nurse and urged her to send drug orders his way (Aikens, 1916, p. 303). Less dependent on the pharmacist than on the physician in 1916, the nurse certainly would have had an easier time coping with him than with the married doctor. Today, the pharmacist may be more problematic because gift giving is such a well established part of commercial relations.

Quality of Nursing Practice in Private Duty

Although nurses in home care had few problems having to do with the obedience of one nurse to another, nurses still had issues regarding the quality of care provided by other private duty nurses. Aikens described a problem of a nurse who is working in home with another nurse who "is careless and does very poor work, is exceedingly disagreeable, and will accept no suggestion as to change" (Aikens, 1916, p. 299). She told a second story of a visiting nurse who, upon finding an old man and woman home sick and desperate, merely took a temperature, gave the wife a bath, and left. Aikens asked, "Did the nurse do her full duty in this case?" Robb recommended that private duty nurses provide each other with the same confidentiality regarding quality of care that they offered physicians. They were not to criticize each other before "either doctor or patient," but a nurse with problems was to be dealt with "privately by her colleagues as a body" and as a last resort, she was to be "publicly dropped from the list of desirable nurses" (Robb, 1901, pp. 259–260).

Current statements of nursing responsibility for the quality of care are, of course, much more direct, and communication among nurses and physicians is improving. Nurses are less dependent on physicians for obtaining cases, and regulations discouraging sexual harassment are at least defined and enforceable in hospitals. However, the stratified structure of health care continues to make the problem of the nurse's role in maintaining quality a continuing one.

RELATIONSHIP TO THE PATIENT

We turn now to what might be considered the key area of nursing ethics, the relationship to the patient. My impression, however, is that so much is devoted in Robb and Aikens to the character of the nurse, relationship to hospital and physicians, economy, etc., that this area gets somewhat short shrift—not that it is unimportant; what is all this dedication to serve except the patient? However, the degree of detail does not measure up to the expression of devotion. In this section, we will discuss the availability of private duty nurses to patients, the role of the nurse as educator in the home, control of care by the patient, and truthfulness with patients and others.

Access of Patients to Private Duty Care

Nurses were obtained for private duty by contacting a variety of registries. Some of these were large and well organized; some were listings kept by schools for alumni; some were small, informal affairs run out of a home. Sometimes many nurses had to be called before one could be found. Many reasons for not seeing patients were regarded as legitimate—vacation, need to rest, illness, waiting on an obstetrical case, etc. Others were not, and nurses came under criticism for being overly selective about cases, lateness, etc. In those prebeeper times, Robb warned nurses to stay close to home when listed as available with the registry and urged nurses not to "spend the day in the country or to do a long morning's shopping" (Robb, 1901, p. 191).

Private duty nurses, like hospital nurses, also specialized in certain types of cases and were able to list limitations on cases with registries. Not only could limitations be expressed in positive, technical terms, but nurses could also, refuse to take certain kinds of cases for a wide range of reasons. In her study, Burgess listed the sorts of practice nurses "registered against" and their frequency:

No limits	39%
Contagion	27%
Obstetrics	18%
Mental	13%
Night	8%
Twenty-four hour	6%
Men	2%
Other	4%

(Burgess, 1928, p. 77)

Contagion is of particular interest ethically because it raises conflicts between the nurse's welfare and the welfare of her clients. It was of particular interest to nurses, partly because twenty-four-hour in-house service exposed nurses to more risks than work in the hospital. For instance, Aikens described a nurse treating a typhoid fever case in an isolated rural home; the bed offered her was a wooden one infested with bedbugs. So, she ordered a new bed for the patient and a cot for herself from a city firm and charged the family for it. Problems developed when the family refused to pay for the items (Aikens, 1916, pp. 268–269). Robb noted that contagion was a much-discussed issue and observed that she had seen many nurses refuse to take contagious patients. She suggested that the frequency of such refusals was attributable to a lack of a code of ethics in nursing and a "lack of comprehension" of nurses' "moral duties as members of a profession." She claimed:

> If a nurse undertakes to do general nursing it is her bounden duty, no less than that of the physician, to take whatever case may come to her. . . . if a nurse declines to go through fear of her own personal safety, there is no excuse for her. . . . she loses the esteem of her co-workers as well as of the physician, and, worse still, her own self-respect. (Robb, 1901, p. 193–195)

In keeping with her appeals to a military model of decorum, she compared the nurse who refuses contagious patients to the soldier who insists on always fighting in the rear. She believed that in most cases, nurses who contracted diseases only had themselves to blame for failing to use proper prophylactic measures. She made these claims in the context of her acceptance of specialization and would not require a nurse, for instance, to accept a contagious case while waiting on an obstetrical one. Despite her strictness, she noted that the period of quarantine for nurses after seeing contagious cases could be financially costly to them; she also believed that nurses who contracted contagious diseases while in service should be cared for at public expense (Robb, 1901, pp. 194–197).

Aikens urged nurses to be either on call or not on call absolutely and not to be charged with picking cases. Like Robb, she accepted specialization but warned against registering against cases, against being unavailable for trivial reasons, and against lateness in responding to cases (Aikens, 1916, pp. 259–263). A less dramatic but characteristic reservation to calling on cases was the reputation of the nurse.

Case 2–15. The Alcoholic Patient

A nurse is called to care for an alcoholic male patient in a hotel in a small town. The patient is vomiting incessantly, and the heart is in exceedingly bad condition. Should a nurse respond to such a call? If so, what general rules of conduct should she be careful to observe while in the hotel? Mention some general rules which nurses should commonly observe when nursing in hotels, whether the patient is male or female. (Aikens, 1916, p. 295)

Actually, this case involves a number of themes. Some nurses refused to work with alcoholic patients or with men patients, although Aikens warned nurses against making moral judgments about patients. Providing care for patients in hospitals was itself common enough that Dietz devoted an entire chapter to the subject (Dietz, 1939, pp. 173–178). Apparently, risk to propriety was a major danger to nurses in these early days. In contrast to today's ethical concerns, none of the texts appear to discuss the personal risks of entering dangerous neighborhoods.

The Nurse as Patient Educator

Education was a major responsibility of the public health nurse from the inception of the field; however, the private duty nurse focused primarily on the care of the sick and less on education. Robb, however, mentioned education as an important role:

> As an educator in the laws of health and right living, the nurse is gradually assuming her proper place, so that people are beginning to rely upon her cooperation to aid in preventing the spread of contagious diseases, by her timely precautions in places where she discovers their existence. By the way in which she does her work in the house in which sickness is present, she can teach the principles of home nursing and certain of the laws of health as regards proper clothing, the best methods of preparing food most suitable to the various conditions existing in health and disease, how to recognize certain adulterations of the more common articles of diet, how to guard against infections, disease, and how to meet emergencies. (Robb, 1901, p. 263)

Since "right living" is included, the nurse was invited to engage in moral education as well. Indeed, the nurse's role as moral educator mirrored the role of nursing educators in preparing nurses for practice. About 1915, a rabbi commented on the image of nurse as moral educator:

> It is easy to state how many visits the nurse makes in the course of a year, how many patients she has seen, but who can tell you to what degree she has reawakened the dormant ambition, or shamed the mother for her slovenliness, or roused a drunken father to a sense of duty to his wife and children. . . . [The visiting nurse] leaves an inspiration to be something a little more and something a little better than they have been. (Franklin, 1984)

Pushing the limits of this conception, Aikens raised the appropriate question as to what extent a nurse should discuss politics and religion with her patient. She also entertained a case where the patient, in a state of repentance after "weeks of social dissipation," wanted to see a minister but the family did not want one called. Aikens wondered what the role of the nurse should be in obtaining a minister to improve the patient's mental condition (Aikens, 1916, p. 302).

Control of Patients and Patient Autonomy

Respect for patient autonomy in the home was definitely qualified in the early years of nursing ethics. Robb expected the private duty nurse to exercise substantial control over the patient:

> Let her determine, then, that the patient's wishes are always worthy of consideration, and that in all nonessentials they should be yielded to, even though they may antagonize her own. On the other hand, when the patient, through ignorance of the real state of affairs, or in the querulousness of sickness, desires something that is opposed to his best interests, it is the nurse's duty to be unyielding, although her authority should be exerted so pleasantly and with such tact and good judgment that neither the patient nor his friends feel that they are being thwarted, but that they are only doing right in following her suggestions. (Robb, 1901, p. 216).

We observe here, as in other cases, that nurses were expected to exercise their power unobtrusively. No intricate discussion of patient consent can be found in this early literature, although the duty of honesty receives some attention.

Truth Telling

Aikens recommended honesty balanced with discreetness. In reporting her own mistakes to supervisors and in reporting the patient's condition to physicians, the nurse should be absolutely honest. Yet, Aikens warned nurses against being too bluntly truthful with a patient who inquires, "Have I got consumption?" Indeed, the presumption was not to disclose: "You are rarely sorry for the things you did not say" (Aikens, 1916, pp. 55–56):

> Endless trouble, untold hours of agony have been caused by the thoughtless habit of some nurse talking with patients about things of which she herself has little real knowledge. (Aikens, 1916, p. 57)

Needless to say, this presumption of silence and discretion also favored keeping information about patients confidential. Aikens reported a scandalous case of leaking information regarding the birth defect of the child of a prominent couple. The problem was traced to a "married nurse who encouraged pupils to bring all the gossip of the hospital to her." She also discouraged nurses from sharing their personal concerns with patients (Aikens, 1916, pp. 58, 128–129). Lounsbery shared the same view: "Never tell revolting hospital stories to your patients. . . .

Never gossip about your sister nurses" (Lounsbery, 1912, pp. 97, 99). Nevertheless, Aikens raised difficult cases in private nursing. In one case, the nurse deceived family and patient in regard to the patient, a suicidally depressed young boy who was being underfed according to medical orders. She fed the boy and he improved markedly. Everyone was pleased, but the nurse was remorseful (Aikens, 1916, p. 293). Another case involved confidentiality in sexually transmitted diseases.

Case 2–16. Gonorrhea

A nurse is called to an obstetrical patient on the second day after the birth of the child. The baby's eyes are infected. The patient, privately to the nurse, blames the doctor, whom she declares was in a great hurry and did not take proper care of her and the child at delivery. The doctor privately tells the nurse that the husband is to blame, that he had previously had gonorrhea and thought himself cured. What should the nurse do when questioned by the patient as to how the infection occurred, and when the patient is telling all her friends that the doctor's neglect is the cause of the trouble? (Aikens, 1916, p. 294)

With the rising rate of AIDS cases, the issues of confidentiality and personal risk are becoming more compelling for nurses. It is fortunate that these questions were raised in the early days of nursing ethics. However, according to the general principles of communication indicated above, what could the nurse do but defend the doctor's reputation and trust that he would handle the problem of the infection discreetly?

SUMMARY

Nurses doing home care today will notice some overlap and similarity between the issues they now face and the issues private duty nurses in the home faced at the turn of the century. They will also notice considerable differences in style and in specific recommendations. Some issues that appeared to be ethics issues then now appear to be merely issues of etiquette. This is probably because we have passed by those questions for the time and now find other issues more difficult. Certainly, recent ethical treatments talk more in terms of general principles and give less concrete advice than do the early nursing ethicists. The "advice" approach certainly suffered from a lack of firm foundations. However, a too-theoretical approach tends to lack specific advice a nurse may need when visiting a home. Let us hope that the new style of ethics will pay off in the long run with both sound foundations and good advice.

Early nursing ethics was also a broader area than ethics is now conceived to be. It included questions of personal health, economy in the home, and the cultural development of nurses. Another way to describe this change is to say that certain distinctions had not yet been made; once made, these distinctions took on a life of their own and led to new areas of special attention. Books on care of the dying, family dynamics, personal relations, community service, and the like cover in more detail concerns merely touched on in the ethics works.

Most strikingly, concern with the qualifications, skills, and competency of nurses has become a field separate from the ethics of the nurse. The "scientific" age of ethics and professionalism in the 1940s to 1950s marked a watershed in which ethics and sciences stepped far apart, as though they were two separate cultures. An indication of this period's effect is that the term "service" and the ideal of service are seldom mentioned in nursing ethics literature. Now, the plural form "services" is used much more often, as a scanning of the Code for Nurses will show (American Nurses' Association, 1985). To use Sandra Harding's term, the ideal of service has been "cooled out" and translated into technical skills and professional or bureaucratic responsibilities (Harding, 1980). Much of the personal quality of the ideal of service has been lost.

Moreover, the recent focus in nursing ethics literature on patient autonomy is misleading. Autonomy is being discussed now, not because we are just recognizing it and permitting more patient control. Instead, we are talking about it more now because patients are losing ground in control over health care. Hospitals are larger and more bound by rules; insurance companies and the federal government have a more substantial role in care. And, the nurse entering the home brings with her now a potential for many social interventions that were not possible in the early days of nursing ethics. For instance, a private duty nurse at the turn of the century would have had little recourse in dealing with suspected child abuse; now he or she must report any suspicions to child protective services. Most important, the home care nurse is employed by an agency, sees several patients, and does not live in the home. All of these factors substantially decrease the control of patient and family over the nurse; the obverse side of this change is that control by patients has decreased.

Homes, hospitals, nursing schools, agencies, and registries have changed a great deal in the last century. Just in terms of technology, the early nursing ethics works were written for homes where much food was grown and even store-bought food was processed extensively, where plumbing and electricity were scarce, where homes were heated by open fires, where clothing and sheets were often made by the woman of the house, etc. A paid visitor to the home was a rarity; now the nurse is one among many people, goods, and equipment that cross the home threshold in a much more consumerist approach to family life. Although these changes have created many liberties, they may be among the forces contributing to the reduction of family size and the increasing instability of the family as an institution. Ironically, as home care is again on the rise, the home is becoming smaller, more unstable, and less protected by privacy and family ties.

The Golden Rule is now for the most part gone from talk of nursing ethics and has been replaced by utilitarianism, formalism, autonomy, beneficence, and justice. The Golden Rule was exhausted by its ambiguities, its incipient paternalism, and its personalization of the professional role. Reputation and propriety are also gone—in our large urban settings where most of our encounters are with strangers, how can anyone ever have a reputation? Fidelity and efficiency are perhaps the prime vocabulary words that remain from the early days of nursing ethics.

The good news is that nursing ethics now serve nurses as professionals and persons more effectively than before. Instead of teaching silence and obedience, they now favor assertiveness, forthrightness, advocacy, excellence, and fairness for professionals and clients alike.

The big questions remain and continue to develop new forms: What is the relationship between the nurse as a person and the nurse in his or her professional capacity? What is the responsibility of professionals and their agencies for each other's actions? Who controls nursing care—nurse, patient, physician, public policy, or the march of history? And most importantly, how can an ideal of service and respect for patients be expressed in work while maintaining respect and equitable rewards for the professional?

REFERENCES

Aikens, C.A. (1916). *Studies in Ethics for Nurses*. Philadelphia: W.B. Saunders Company.

Aikens, C.A. (1943). *Studies in Ethics for Nurses* (5th ed.). Philadelphia: W.B. Saunders Company.

American Journal of Nursing. (1927). Ethical problems: Problem VII. *American Journal of Nursing, 27*:372.

American Journal of Nursing. (1931). Ethical problems: Problem V. *American Journal of Nursing, 31*:493.

American Nurses' Association. (1985). *Code for Nurses with Interpretive Statements*. Kansas City, MO: American Nurses' Association.

Ashley, J.A. (1976). *Hospitals, Paternalism, and the Role of the Nurse*. New York: Teachers College Press.

Ashley, J.A. (1975). Nurses in American history: Nursing and early feminism. *American Journal of Nursing, 75*:1465–1467.

Bermosk, L.S., & Corsini, R.J. (Eds.). (1973). *Critical Incidents in Nursing.* Philadelphia: W.B. Saunders Company.

Burgess, M.A. (1926). Five rules for diagram making. *American Journal of Nursing, 26*:675.

Burgess, M.A. (1928). *Nurses, Patient, and Pocketbooks: Report of a Study of the Economics of Nursing Conducted by the Committee on the Grading of Nursing Schools.* New York: Committee on the Grading of Nursing Schools.

Densford, K.J., and Everett, M.S. (1947). *Ethics for Modern Nurses: Professional Adjustments. Vol. 1.* Philadelphia: W.B. Saunders Company.

Dietz, L.D. (1939). *Professional Problems of Nurses* (3rd ed.). Philadelphia: F.A. Davis Co.

Edgell, B. (1929). *Ethical Problems: An Introduction to Ethics for Hospital Nurses and Social Workers.* London: Methuen & Co. Ltd.

Fowler, M.D. (1984). *Ethics and Nursing, 1893–1984: The Ideal of Service, the Reality of History.* University of Southern California.

Franklin, L. (1984, April 18). *Omaha Visiting Nurse Association Centenary Program*, Omaha, Nebraska.

Goodhart, A.L. (1938). Hospitals and trained nurses. *Law Quarterly Review, 54*:553–575.

Harding, S. (1980). Value-laden technologies and the politics of nursing. In S.F. Spicker & S. Gadow (Eds.), *Nursing: Images and Ideals: Opening Dialogue with the Humanities* (pp. 49–75). New York: Springer Publishing Company.

Huggett, F.E. (1977). *Life Below Stairs: Domestic Servants in England from Victorian Times.* London: John Murray.

Kelly, L.Y. (1981). *Dimensions of Professional Nursing* (4th ed.). New York: Macmillan Publishing Company.

Lounsbery, H.C. (1912). *Making Good on Private Duty: Practical Hints to Graduate Nurses.* Philadelphia: J.B. Lippincott Company.

Martin, L., & Segrave, K. (1985). *The Servant Problem: Domestic Workers in North America.* Jefferson, NC: McFarland & Company, Inc.

Moore, J. (1988). *A Zeal for Responsibility: The Struggle for Professional Nursing in Victorian England, 1868–1883.* Athens, GA: The University of Georgia Press.

The open forum: Two puzzling questions. (1934). *American Journal of Nursing, 34*:1010.

Parsons, S.E. (1916). *Nursing Problems and Obligations.* Boston: Whitcomb & Barrows.

Reverby, S.M. (1987). *Ordered to Care: The Dilemma of American Nursing, 1850–1945.* Cambridge: Cambridge University Press.

Robb, I.H. (1901). *Nursing Ethics: For Hospital and Private Use.* Cleveland: J.B. Savage.

Spalding, E.K. (1939). *Professional Adjustments in Nursing: For Senior Students and Graduates.* Philadelphia: J.B. Lippincott Company.

Thompson, H.S. (1905). Ethics in private practice. *American Journal of Nursing, 6*:163–166.

Chapter 3

Ethical Issues in the Care of Clients and Their Families

Amy Marie Haddad

Ethical decision making is a cognitive process. It requires knowledge of ethical principles, traditions, theories, and sound clinical and situational data. However, ethical problems in practice are not clear cut. They involve personalities, motivations, perceptions and opinions. In other words, they involve human beings with all of their complexity and diversity. The following case study illustrates the interpersonal dynamics that make sound ethical decision making a challenge.

Case 3–1. Client versus Staff Beneficence

On January 16, Jane Langely was admitted to the pulmonary intensive care unit of Northeast General Hospital after sustaining severe burns (partial- and full-thickness burns to her arms, trunk, and neck) and severe damage to both lungs due to inhalation burns. Jane, 24, was a college student. She was injured in a house fire after a "wild party," according to friends who had been at the party. She had fallen asleep on the couch and woke in the midst of the fire.

After several months in the pulmonary intensive care unit, it is apparent that Jane will be ventilator-dependent for the rest of her life. "Her lungs are like those of a 60-year-old with chronic pulmonary disease," her primary physician, Dr. Abraham, commented. "The smoke inhalation, the high oxygen settings, and the ventilator pressures have all caused permanent damage."

Approximately 1 year after her admission, Dr. Abraham began to discuss discharge. Dr. Abraham told the discharge planner, "Jane has reached a plateau. There is nothing more that we can do for her here." Jane's father's insurance carrier will cover acute care for Jane as long as necessary, so there is no economic pressure to move her. Yet Dr. Abraham is adamant about moving Jane out of the hospital. Mr. and Mrs. Langely agree to move Jane to their home. Dr. Abraham writes the orders for twenty-four-hour-per-day skilled nursing care for thirty days. Dr. Abraham told the charge nurse, "I'm sure Jane and the Langelys can handle her care after a month. The home care agency can reinforce the teaching we've begun here."

The discharge is planned for the following week. Jane and her parents have been taught to perform tracheostomy care and some other basic skills. The durable medical equipment supplier brought in the ventilator that Jane will use at home, so she could adjust to it before discharge. Jane and her parents have never changed the circuits on the ventilator nor changed Jane's tracheostomy tube.

Your home care agency has been selected to provide care for Jane after discharge. In preparing for the discharge, you discuss Jane's care with the following people: Jane, her parents, staff nurses, the physician, the occupational, physical, and recreational therapists, the dietitian, and the social worker. From these encounters, you begin to piece together a more complete picture of Jane. Jane had been on her own for the previous five years before the accident occurred. She had always been very independent and reluctant to commit herself to the rigidity of a career or college. She worked odd jobs, traveled around the country with a group of "bikers," and generally lived a free and easy life, taking each day as it came. Her parents did not approve of her life-style or her friends. Contact between Jane and her parents before the accident was minimal and strained.

VALUES, RIGHTS, AND RESPONSIBILITIES

A complex, high-tech home care case, such as the one described in the case study, is replete with challenges for the home care agency. These challenges include the organization of technically competent staff, the development of a workable plan of care, and discussions with the client and family about expectations of home care. The case study also presents significant ethical challenges that are not as immediately apparent. The case is representative of those frequently encountered in home care and will serve as a focus for the discussion of key ethical principles and philosophical questions in the care of clients and their families.

An examination of the ethical issues in the case study, and by extension real-life ethical problems, requires an understanding of ethical principles, theories, and the specific ethical obligations of home care providers. It also requires an appreciation of the personalities, motivations, perceptions and opinions of those involved (Salladay & Haddad, 1986). Therefore, one of the most important aspects of ethical analysis is strictly descriptive: What is going on here (Post, 1987)?

The trauma that Jane has undergone is both physical and psychological. As such it necessitates both physical and psychological healing (Mattsson, 1975). Jane's physical healing processes have received a great deal of professional attention. Psychological healing processes, though recognized, have remained in the background. Jane is a product of our technologically sophisticated health care system. It has given life to Jane but left her in a condition of relative dependence on family and professional caregivers.

There is a pluralism of principles at work in the case study. Each individual has rights and responsibilities. "A right is a justified claim or claims that individuals or groups can make upon others or upon society" (Beauchamp & Childress, 1983, p. 50). Jane's right to adequate care, her family's right to privacy, and the home care agency's right to information regarding Jane's case are all legitimate rights and yet may be in conflict.

The responsibilities of the principals involved are numerous and diverse. Responsibility implies chargeability, in that an individual is answerable to something in their control or power (Allen, 1974). There are many "senses" of responsibility, but in home care, the emphasis is more likely to be on role-responsibility. Role-responsibility recognizes the fact that there are distinctive places in social life that carry with them certain duties and obligations. These are the responsibilities of the role. "But the responsibilities go beyond specific duties and obligations. They define a sphere of concern, which usually cannot be delimited in finite, specifiable ways" (Dworkin, 1981, p. 27). Since Jane has not been close to her family for the last several years, her role is indistinct. The role of "daughter" may not carry with it any clear obligations in the Langely family. Likewise, the Langelys' interpretation of the role of "parent" and its corresponding duties may be outdated as the Langelys must now deal with a competent, adult–child. The Langelys are not unique in their role confusion. Illness and injury often bring about alterations in family roles.

The case raises a number of ethical questions regarding responsibility: What obligations do parents have to adult children? What responsibilities does the home care agency assume when they agree to take a client like Jane home? What are Jane's responsibilities, if any, as the recipient of care?

The ascribing of rights and responsibilities is predicated on the value systems of those involved. Values are those deeply held beliefs or attitudes that define what an individual thinks is important. Each of the individuals involved in the case study have values regarding their expectations of home care. Therefore, the first step in examining the ethical implications of Jane's care is to consider the values of Jane, her parents, and the home care provider.

Client's Perspective and Values

It is difficult to categorize Jane's primary problem. On the one hand, Jane is the victim of a traumatic injury, a severe burn. The fire and its sequelae can be viewed as a crisis. Therefore, care delivery could focus on the adaptive tasks encountered in managing a crisis. On the other hand, Jane has a chronic illness. She essentially has chronic obstructive pulmonary disease secondary to her burn injury. Therefore, care delivery could focus on the adaptive tasks encountered in living with a chronic illness. Finally, Jane could be considered terminally ill. The damage to her lungs is irreversible and progressive, which will eventually result in a pneumothorax or respiratory arrest.

Therefore, even the development of the plan of care has ethical implications in that the formulation of the primary problem and subsequent treatment protocols are shaped by the values of the home care personnel involved. These values are further shaped by various psychological factors, one of which is primary effect, or more commonly, first impressions related to a client, his or her diagnosis, and care needs. There is a strong tendency to value information that is learned first (Salladay & Haddad, 1986). If, for example, Jane is initially presented to the home care provider as a terminally ill client, it will be difficult, later on, to discount this view.

These distinctions are not superfluous. There are clear expectations and goals associated with each perspective. It is essential to Jane's care for those involved to understand the personal meaning she gives to her health status and present situation. The lack of congruence between the client's, parents', and home care providers' perceptions can be a source of conflict unless those involved are able to communicate and negotiate a common perspective on the problem (Stuifbergen, 1987).

Jane may feel overpowered by her physical limitations. At the same time, it may be very difficult for her to accept comfort and support when these are most necessary. Jane's condition requires a total readjustment in every facet of her life. Central to this readjustment is the somatic assault of the ventilator (Lambert & Lambert, 1987). Incorporation of the ventilator as part of oneself is not uncommon in ventilator patients. The ventilator dictates whether Jane lives or dies so she must contend with the control of the machine.

In addition to adjusting to alterations in bodily appearance resulting from the burn scarring and the ventilator, Jane is also being required to: (1) manage complicated health care regimens; (2) deal with symptoms and their meanings; (3) handle the uncertainty of the progression of the disease; and (4) revise personal and social goals (Lambert & Lambert, 1987). Though Jane has the right to be involved in her care and discharge planning, she may not have the will or energy to participate.

Jane, like all hospitalized patients, has forfeited a great deal of her independence and has submitted to the dependent role created for her in the hospital. The traditional attitude toward patient responsibilities was largely defined by Parsons (1951), who theorized that the sick role was composed of certain behaviors, which included exemption from usual role tasks and responsibilities. Though this model is useful for examining the role responsibilities of acutely ill clients with distinct periods of illness and recovery, it is not helpful in examining the role responsibilities of the chronically ill.

Because of these limitations, arguments in favor of attributing responsibilities to clients have been put forward by others (Jameton, 1988; Kelly & May, 1982; Tagliaczzo & Mauksch, 1979). "For the most part, patients are able to meet responsibilities, and most sickness is limited enough to permit relatively full lives" (Jameton, 1988). Thus, even though Jane is limited in her ability to assume responsibilities, it is preferable to assess what she is able to do and wants to assume rather than sweepingly eliminate responsibilities altogether (Jameton, 1988).

Family's Perspective and Values

Mr. and Mrs. Langely are middle-aged adults faced with the responsibility of an adult-child to whom they have not been close for many years. Their past relationship with Jane does have a bearing on their rights and responsibilities in the case. Unfortunately, little attention has been given to prior functioning or the process aspects of family relationships (eg, communication) that may account for differences in family adaptation to illness, chronic or otherwise (Stuifbergen, 1987).

Regardless of the quality of the Langely's past relationship with their daughter, there is a certain degree of familial obligation at work in the case. Parents are expected to care for their children. "Breaches of faithfulness in the family are viewed with special disdain because loyalty and moral idealism, although far from the normative in the wider society, are considered necessary for the family's common life" (Post, 1987, p. 57). Family loyalties should be constant despite the strains that necessarily arise in complex home care. This value is evident in Mr. Langely's comments, "We're Jane's parents. We'll take care of her. That's what parents are supposed to do."

Though Mr. and Mrs. Langely may have an obligation to care, in the sense of loving their daughter, it does not follow that they have an obligation to personally deliver the care or even provide space in their home for Jane. It would be important to determine if any other options were presented to the Langelys when they agreed to take Jane into their home. Were alternative living accommodations recommended or available? It is also important to determine the time frame in which the Langelys have placed their responsibility. Do they feel obligated to provide a home for Jane until she can manage her own care? Or are they taking her home for the duration, however long that may be?

The Langelys are at a developmental stage where they are beginning to enjoy the fruits of their labors. Their obligations for childrearing had seemingly ended. Both of them are highly involved in their work. Mrs. Langely returned to a career in accounting five years ago and is just now gaining a position of authority in a job she loves. Jane's return into their lives has been disruptive and unsettling.

Home Care Providers' Perspectives and Values

Though conflicts have not arisen yet, there is the potential for conflicts about the desired ends to be gained by home care. Two goals have already been established for home care: (1) Jane and her parents will become proficient in basic respiratory care; and (2) Jane and her family will take responsibility for Jane's care in a month. Certain assumptions have been taken for granted regarding the end to be pursued. Conflicts arise when these ends have not been examined by all those involved. For example, Dr. Abraham has established the aforementioned goals based on the assumption that "Jane and the Langelys can handle her care after a month." This is a questionable assumption as Jane and her parents have not demonstrated a desire to work toward this end in the hospital. It is doubtful their behavior will change when Jane goes home.

The previously mentioned assumption reflects two commonly held values regarding rehabilitation of disabled persons. The first unspoken value is that family participation is expected and an important factor in Jane's rehabilitation. Watson (1987) examined the value of family participation from the perspective of rehabilitators. The findings indicated that rehabilitators valued family participation and, in contrast to the current literature in rehabilitation, believed in a directive model in which the family defers to the wishes of the health care providers (Watson, 1987).

Second, there is an implied value in working toward independence. According to this value, those involved in Jane's care should encourage her to ". . . function at a maximum level of independence and to engage, as soon as possible, in the regular performance of family duties and leisure activities" (Power, 1989, p. 74).

Most home care agencies place a high value on their ability to provide good care. This value is actualized in the expertise of their personnel, attention to quality, and most concretely, in the home care agency's standards of care. The standards of care provide a quantitative and qualitative measure of the home care agency's basic responsibilities to the client. It is apparent that Jane has not always complied with accepted standards of care regarding her respiratory hygiene in the hospital. The home care agency could anticipate that its responsibility to provide quality care for Jane may conflict with her right to determine her treatment.

To provide quality care for all clients with whom the home care agency has a contract, it is also its responsibility to initiate the discussions that will bring about an agreement regarding the goals, or ends, of home care. The first step in this process is the clarification of these values by all concerned. In all cases, there is a hierarchy of values that each individual holds that, at least, must be partially reconciled in order for rights to be honored and responsibilities fulfilled.

Case 3–1A. Working Toward Discharge

In the hospital, Jane was fundamentally uninvolved in her care. She claimed to be too weak or too tired to assist and so the nurses ended up completing the care. Jane quickly learned how to suction herself but reluctantly followed through with the task and only after much coaxing and pushing by the nursing staff. She halfheartedly worked with the physical therapist and walked short distances down the hall from her room. The occupational therapist was at the end of her patience with Jane. Jane completely refused to cooperate with any of the occupational therapist's suggestions. The dietician finally quit arguing with Jane regarding her diet. The dietician had increased the gastrostomy feedings to make up for the calories Jane wasn't taking orally. The dietician suggested that the home care agency might have better luck getting Jane to eat at home as the ultimate treatment goal was to get her off gastrostomy feedings entirely.

The social worker had extensive experience in working with burn patients. She commented, "Burns, like almost all accidental injuries, happen with far greater frequency to people under stress in the first place. Almost any type of burn points a statistical arrow at a group under stress: the poor, the alcohol- and drug-addicted, the mentally ill, the unemployed. People like this have a difficult enough time handling ordinary problems in life. The obstacles of a major burn will be difficult for Jane to overcome. Her premorbid coping was poor. I expect that she will have serious psychiatric problems that just haven't surfaced yet" (Tisdale, 1986).

The practice of home care is a meeting between two parties, one seeking help and the other offering it. The meeting has serious implications for those involved. "Such a meeting imposes stringent moral demands on both parties; it requires trust, honesty, cooperation, competence, and compassion" (Jonsen, Siegler, & Winslade, 1982, p. 3). These virtues arise from the ethical principles of respect for persons and beneficence. Since the initial contact between home care provider and client primarily involves these two principles, they will be examined in detail in relation to the case study. This section first examines autonomy and its corollary, informed consent.

Autonomy and Informed Consent

A key component of the discharge planning process is the involvement of the client and family in the planning. Dennis (1987) identified activities that give patients a sense of control during hospitalization. The following activities were important to hospitalized adults for getting well or going home.

> Very important to patients was knowing whether their condition was improving or deteriorating, understanding what the diagnosis meant to their way of life in general, and knowing which physical activities were restricted. (Dennis, 1987, p. 153)

Having information about these factors was critical to clients' development of cognitive control.

This information sharing is a form of informed consent. Obtaining consent for treatment, in this case home care, is a legal and ethical obligation. "Ethically valid consent is a process of shared decision making based upon mutual respect and participation, not a ritual to be equated with reciting the contents of a form that details the risks of particular treatments" (President's Commission for the Study of Ethical Problems in Medicine and Biomedical and Behavioral Research, 1983, p. 20).

Since the home care provider is not asking for consent to a specific treatment or procedure, the whole process of obtaining consent is less well defined. In its original intent, the doctrine of informed consent applied to acutely ill patients with discrete health care needs for which there is a specific course of medical treatment. Home care does not generally deal with acute episodes of illness so the traditional model of informed consent must be adapted for home care.

Home care takes place in a different environment from acute care and usually extends over a longer period of time. This allows more time to inform individuals about their condition and to develop the plan of care. The home care provider sees the client and the family in a more realistic light than health care providers in the acute care setting. "The full impact of the illness or injury is normally not realized in the artificial, controlled environment of the hospital. Most of the client's and family's social, emotional, and environmental adjustment occurs after the return home to the reality of daily living" (Haddad, 1987, p. 137–138).

Since home care is not usually delivered in the urgent manner of acute care and can therefore be undertaken at a relatively slower pace, informed consent should flourish in the context of the home environment (Cohen, 1987). However, two factors may make informed consent more difficult in the home care setting. First of all, it is very difficult to predict what will actually occur after the client returns home. Even the most detailed discharge plan cannot foresee the complications that may arise in the home.

Second, it is clearly one thing to get a client to sign a permit for a cholecystectomy and another to sign an agreement to provide home care. Consent evolves over time in home care and involves more than just the client. Therefore, informed consent becomes a process rather than a discrete event and is complicated by the involvement of family members, friends and others who are part of the client's home life.

The doctrine of informed consent is the legal mechanism by which patient autonomy is protected (Youngner, 1986, p. 42). "Autonomy is that quality which describes the degree of mastery an individual exercises over his or her life" (Cohen, 1985). The concept of autonomy is tied to the ideas of self-determination, self-responsibility, freedom, privacy, and independence.

Respect for autonomy is the obligation not to interfere with the choice of another and to treat another as being capable of choosing (Miller, 1981). Individuals have a right to plan their own lives in a way they see fit. However, individuals do not act in isolation. "Autonomy is not limited to the impact on oneself, for surely autonomy and its exercise clearly have an impact on others" (Cohen, 1985). Thus, the home care agency has an obligation to respect Jane's autonomy and perhaps to encourage her to assert her ownership of what happens to her. On the other hand, the home care agency must also examine the impact Jane's decisions have on others.

Necessary Conditions of Autonomy. Faden and Beauchamp (1986, p. 238) make the assumption that the following conditions are necessary for an autonomous action: "X acts autonomously only if X acts (1) intentionally; (2) with understanding; and (3) without controlling influences." An autonomous action, like informed consent, requires sufficient understanding. The individual must have an understanding of his or her own action. Though there are various interpretations of what "understanding" means in the context of informed decision making in health care, it typically means that patients come to understand *that* they must consent to or refuse a particular proposal by understanding *what* is communicated in an informational exchange with a professional (Faden & Beauchamp, 1986, p. 250).

Does Jane understand what has been communicated to her by the various health care professionals involved? Further, does she understand the consequences of her decisions? Even though it is extremely difficult to measure the extent of an individual's understanding, an attempt should be made to determine if Jane can correctly describe the nature of the action (eg, "I don't want to eat anything by mouth"), and the foreseeable consequences and outcomes of performing or not performing the action (eg, "If I don't eat anything by mouth, I will be completely dependent on the gastrostomy feedings for nourishment").

Finally, an autonomous action is free from coercion or undue external influence. Is Jane being pressured to act in a certain way? In Jane's case, it appears that the health care professionals involved have been doing their best to persuade Jane to participate in her care with no success. In fact, some of the health care professionals have resorted to coercion in order to get Jane to comply with treatment protocols. For example, the physical therapist often withheld Jane's right to have visitors until Jane completed her exercises. He justified his action by noting, "That was the only way I could get her to cooperate."

Another factor that influences Jane's ability to make an autonomous decision is the presence of a severe injury and ongoing physiological insult. Jackson and Youngner (1979) studied the decisions of patients in an intensive care unit and concluded that little "true autonomy" is to be found in the choices of the patients. Many of the patients were depressed, overwhelmed by their injuries and symptoms, and deeply ambivalent about their treatment.

Senses of Autonomy. In addition to the necessary conditions for autonomous action cited by Faden and Beauchamp (1986), Miller (1981) has proposed several senses of the concept of autonomy. An action does not necessarily merit respect merely because it is authentic or the result of effective deliberation. But an examination of the senses of autonomy can illuminate the problem of whether one is obliged to honor or override another's autonomy.

Autonomy can be viewed as free action. Autonomy in this sense includes the condition of freedom from undue control previously discussed. No action can be completely free. Therefore, actions are considered to be substantially free, taking into account the numerous factors that influence all of our decisions.

Autonomy as authenticity "means that an action is consistent with the person's attitudes, values, dispositions, and life plans. Roughly, the person is acting in character" (Miller, 1981, p. 24).

Is Jane acting in character? Would we expect her to accept treatment recommendations or refuse them? More basically, how has Jane normally responded to authority figures and their recommendations? The family could also be asked to offer an opinion on whether a patient is acting as he would normally act, or whether his or her behavior strikes them as aberrant or unusual (Siegler, 1977). When asked, Mrs. Langely commented, "Jane has always done the opposite thing. No matter what I tell her she will go out of her way to do the exact opposite." Mr. Langely concurred, "Jane has always been headstrong, just like her mother." In Jane's case, her actions appear to be authentic and yet work against her best interest; for example, if she refuses to walk and remains inactive, she stands a good chance of getting a respiratory infection.

Autonomy as effective deliberation means action taken after weighing the consequences of alternatives in a situation calling for a decision and choosing an action based on that evaluation (Miller, 1981). Effective deliberation is not present when an individual acts impulsively. Jane may have effectively deliberated on the alternatives available to her and chosen the one that required the least amount of energy. Persons afflicted with chronic obstructive pulmonary disease may find that simply confronting a change in emotion, be it happy or sad, or physical activity, such as eating, walking, upper body exercises, can rapidly upset the precarious cardiopulmonary system, with the end result being respiratory imbalance and distress (Dudley, Glaser, Jorgenson, & Lagan, 1980).

Jane's actions may be the result of effective deliberation regarding the very real precariousness of her physiological status and the risks she is willing to take in disrupting it. However, Jane may not fully appreciate the long-term implications of the alternatives she has chosen. Rational deliberation does not always yield right results. "Right results are not an essential concomitant of autonomous action" (Cohen, 1985, p. 146). The home care provider has an obligation to return to areas of disagreement in treatment procedures that act against the client's long-term interests as the home care provider interprets them.

Jane's noncompliance or unwillingness to follow through with the recommendations of the health care professionals involved in her case could also be due to her desire to regain her independence. Noncompliance may be seen as an aspect of her struggles not to let her injury take undue control of her life; in this sense, it supports her desires for independence and autonomy, desires that align closely with the therapeutic goals of her caregivers (Conrad, 1987). Taken from this perspective, Jane may not conceive of her behavior as noncompliant.

Internal Problems of Autonomy. The discussion of autonomy to this point has dealt with those factors that should be considered in determining if an action is substantially autonomous. Yet it is not the obvious denial or overriding of self-determination that is so troubling in home care. The subtle erosion of autonomy in small matters may give way to larger matters over time or with increasing chronicity and concomitant dependence on others.

Most decisions in home care are not dramatic life-and-death choices. Collopy (1988) has identified a series of internal tensions in autonomy in the long-term care setting that are equally applicable to home care. These internal polarities include: (1) decisional versus executional; (2) competent versus incapacitated; and (3) immediate versus long-range freedom (Collopy, 1988).

Full autonomy includes both decisional and executional autonomy, that is, the ability to decide on an action and the ability to carry it out. If one is unable to carry out an action because of a physical disability, for example, shouldn't one retain the right to decide? This question is even more pertinent in home care because of the environment. Who is in charge in the home care setting? "In fact, as the outward reach of autonomy shrinks, its inner decisional core becomes a last and therefore most crucial preserve of self-determination" (Collopy, 1988, p. 12). It is a small step to move from feeding a client to deciding what and when he or she will eat.

Jane's decisional autonomy may have already suffered from her year-long hospitalization. It is up to the home care provider to clearly distinguish its role as executor and Jane's role as decision maker.

The competent-versus-incapacitated polarity within autonomy involves a judgment about the rationality of choices. How do we draw the line between competent and incompetent? The following criteria can be used to determine competency. First, can the client make and express choices about life? Second, are the outcomes of the choices reasonable? Third, are the choices based on rational reasons? These three criteria often raise additional questions such as: Reasonable to whom? Rational from whose perspective? One method of determining the rationality of choices is to see if there is a logical consistency. For example, if a client refused to have a gangrenous leg amputated and yet expressed a strong desire to live, this would not be rational.

Finally, the client has to be able to understand the implications of the choices made. So far, Jane's competency has not been called into question. This may be due to the fact that Jane has grudgingly cooperated with treatment and none of her refusals have been taken too seriously. If in the future, however, Jane clearly refuses treatment that the home care provider thinks is in her best interest, her competency might be questioned. Incompetence is one of the few justifications for overriding a client's right to determine what should or should not be done to and for him by another.

> Should a person be unable to comprehend and to act for himself, the legal system specifies various alternatives. A parent or guardian can make decisions on behalf of child or a mentally incompetent person for whom he is responsible. (Kravitz, 1985, p. 34A)

A final area of internal tension exists between respecting the client's autonomy in the present instance or enabling future long-term freedom. These two conditions are not necessarily coherent. If the home care providers respect Jane's present autonomous decision to limit suctioning and circuit changes, are they acting against her future autonomy by complying with this choice? Her immediate freedom may work against her long-range care. The home care provider must decide what is more important, short-term expressions of autonomy or long-range freedoms (Collopy, 1988).

This discussion of the various facets of autonomy serves to reinforce the conclusion that it is no simple matter to determine autonomous and nonautonomous action. The home care provider does not have to respect an action merely because it is autonomous. The object of respect is the *fact* that the other is autonomous (Beauchamp, 1986). This attention to the principle of autonomy is necessary to prevent unnecessary depersonalization, to protect the individuality of clients, and to recognize freedom. However, the idea of autonomy often places the individual in a moral vacuum. Autonomy alone does not help home care providers understand the extent of their obligations to clients. An understanding of the principle of beneficence is necessary if we are to fully appreciate our obligations to one another.

Duty of Beneficence

The term "beneficence" has many meanings and may include the duty not to harm as well as the more positive obligations to help others. "In its most general form, the principle of beneficence requires us to abstain from injuring others and to help others further their important or legitimate interests, largely by preventing or removing possible harms" (Beauchamp & Walters, 1982, p. 28). Most duties of beneficence, the positive assistance to others, derive from roles and commitments, such as those a home care provider undertakes with a client. Often in health care there is a fine line between helping others, remaining indifferent, and harming.

Beneficence is at the heart of the home care provider's commitment to care. This basic dictum to be compassionate, humane, and caring toward those for whom we provide care is most often expressed in the phrase "to treat the whole person." This is especially true in the context of home care where the health care provider is allowed to see the client and family in their own environment.

To be concerned with the "whole person" and to practice with consideration and sensitivity for the integrity of the human self is basically an ethical injunction (Zaner, 1974). In a caring relationship, "one experiences what is cared for as having a dignity and worth in its own right with potentialities and need for growth. Caring is the antithesis of possessing, manipulating, or dominating, a process which requires devotion and trust" (Carper, 1986, p. 4). The concepts of respect for persons and caring are intertwined and inseparable.

The home care providers must balance their obligations to care for the client with the client's autonomy. "Even patients who are competent can exert poor judgment when they are ill or injured, and a crisis arises if they will not consent to proposed treatment" (Beauchamp & Walters, 1982, p. 30). The home care providers must decide if they are going to accept the client's refusal as valid, and thus respect the client's autonomy, or override the client's decision in order to benefit the client. The problem of whether to override the decisions of clients to benefit them is obvious in the case study, particularly after Jane's discharge to her parents' home.

CONFLICT BETWEEN AUTONOMY AND BENEFICENCE

Case 3–1B. Resolving Conflicts

Three weeks after Jane's discharge, the nurses on the case decide that a care conference is in order. Jane has become distant and uninterested in the majority of her care procedures. She refuses to leave her room or even attempt to walk as she gets exhausted. Sometimes it takes an entire shift to get her tracheostomy changed and the circuits changed on her ventilator. Jane is constantly readjusting the ventilator settings from those ordered by Dr. Abraham. Jane is very suspicious of new staff members and makes them go through suctioning technique with one of her regular nurses before she'll let them suction her alone.

Mr. and Mrs. Langely are furious with Jane's lack of participation in her own care. On the other hand, they refuse to participate in any of her care. If the ventilator alarm goes off while Mrs. Langely is in the room alone with Jane, she runs from the room to get the nurse. The primary nurse on the case has asked the Langelys if they would like to learn more about Jane's care. Mr. Langely replied, "I guess in a pinch I would help out with Jane's care but, I'm not always around." Mrs. Langely was clearer about her feelings, "I don't want to touch that machine of hers. It scares me to death. Why, I could cut off her air or something. I don't want anything to do with it."

The deadline Dr. Abraham set for the termination of skilled care is only one week away. Obviously, Jane and the Langelys are not ready for the sole responsibility of Jane's care.

Analyzing the Conflict

The home care provider is in the business of caring for clients, that is, doing good for clients. This obligation to do good is an obligation based on the special knowledge and expertise of the home care provider. Jane has refused to follow a prescribed treatment regimen that the experts (physician, nurses, and other therapists) feel is in her best interest. The home care providers could agree with Jane's decisions and only perform those treatments that she allows, when she allows them. Does this relieve the home care provider of responsibility for Jane's welfare?

Does respect for autonomy mean that we are not allowed to act on the good that we know will benefit another? The home care provider is not only allowed to imagine a good for Jane beyond that which she can imagine for herself but is obligated to persuade Jane to comply with treatment that will help her.

Persuasion is an effort to persuade a change in action or attitude by an appeal to reason; an attempt to induce a person to freely accept a course of action. Persuasion differs from coercion in that coercion is morally unacceptable. Coercion occurs if one party intentionally and successfully influences another by presenting a credible threat of unwanted or unavoidable harm so severe that the person is unable to resist acting to avoid it (Faden & Beauchamp, 1987). Coercion can be legal, economic, physical, or psychological.

The home care provider must determine which components of care are worth persuading the client to change or reconsider. For example, Jane refused to take a shower daily. This became a point of great contention with some of the nurses. In weighing out the relative significance of respecting Jane's autonomy in the area of hygiene, it did not seem as important or life-threatening as suctioning or changing the ventilator circuits. The home care provider must be clear about the issue in conflict. The issue may not be as simple as "to suction or not to suction." The issue may be one of control. Clients with chronic obstructive pulmonary disease often carry out daily respiratory hygiene techniques in a precise and systematic manner. This may be one way for Jane to place stringent controls on her environment. "By placing controls on the environment, they believe they are less likely to encounter an emotionally charged situation that can lead to an emotional upset and subsequent respiratory imbalance" (Lambert & Lambert, 1987, p. 528).

Another explanation for Jane's behavior may be a response to a lack of privacy. Though Jane had adjusted to the lack of privacy in the hospital, it is an entirely different situation now that she is at home. Jane is now in familiar surroundings and the presence of strangers is much more obvious and unsettling. Jane might feel that she is constantly being observed. Since her privacy is so compromised, she might be trying to gain some personal space by avoiding activities, such as her shower, that literally increase her exposure. Protecting privacy is the most fundamental exercise of autonomy.

Therefore, the home care provider is obligated to sort out the components of the conflict, determine underlying motivations, and decide which areas are truly harmful, a matter of aesthetics, or negotiable.

Persuasion does not always change behavior and the home care providers might easily find themselves in a situation where the client's autonomy is clearly in conflict with the home care providers' duty to do good. For example, if Jane persisted in refusal of treatments to the extent that there would be life-threatening consequences and if she appeared to be incapacitated because of her physical status, the home care provider might not only be justified in overriding Jane's wishes, but also morally obligated to do so.

This type of action is known as paternalism. The intention of paternalism is to do good, to benefit another. The consequences of paternalism are to override or ignore the other's wishes. In this case, the home care provider decides for Jane what is in her best interest. Paternalism has further been described as strong or limited according to the decision-making capabilities of the person making the choice.

Childress (1982) has proposed the following guidelines for limited paternalism:

> In limited paternalism, agents meet the needs of other persons without insulting them. For example, if another person is incompetent to make decisions and is also at risk, interventions even against that person's express wishes do not signify disrespect or constitute an indignity. Not to intervene might even violate the principle of respect for persons; certainly, it would violate the principle of beneficence in some circumstances. (Childress, 1982, p. 103)

Both conditions, incompetence and the threat of great harm, must be present to justify limited paternalism. The burden of proof that paternalism is justified rests entirely on those, in this case the home care providers, who propose paternalistic actions because the consent of the person whose liberty is being restricted is not sought (Fromer, 1981).

Working with an Uncooperative Client

Jane's unwillingness to cooperate with the treatment plan triggered a host of negative responses from the nurses assigned to her case. One of the nurses asked to be changed to another case. She stated, "There is a limit as to how much Jane can get away with. I won't stand by and watch her get a respiratory infection because she doesn't like to be suctioned."

This nurse expressed emotions that have been identified in the literature as early as 1957 by Highley and Norris. Nursing students were asked to identify what they disliked in patients. The students' list of dislikes included: "Patients who won't do what the nurse asks them to; won't cooperate; won't obey the rules" (Highley & Norris, 1957, p. 1163).

It is common for caregivers to remove themselves from the care of uncooperative clients. Keller (1971) noted that in the long term, the compliant patient received more services, but in the short term, the noncompliant patient received more services. The caregiver spent more time in the short run trying to ascertain reasons for noncompliant behavior and to persuade the client to cooperate. After it became clear that the client's noncompliance was not amenable to change, the caregivers spent far less time with the client (Keller, 1971).

Kelly and May (1982) defined a good patient as one who confirms the role of the nurse; the bad patient denies that legitimation. Jane has not cooperated with the nurses' attempts to provide care for her. She has also not been grateful or appreciated the benefits extended by the staff. This type of behavior on the part of the client elicits strong emotional responses from the staff that commonly include anger and frustration (Podrasky & Sexton, 1988).

Though this discussion may appear tangential to the principle of beneficence, it is difficult to do good for someone who will not cooperate. Podrasky & Sexton (1988) noted in their study of nurses' reactions to difficult patients that nurses most often reacted behaviorally with a classical fight or flight response rather than seeking to determine the reason for the negative behavior. At times the fight response was manifested as potentially hostile acts or impulses toward patients or by taking anger out with a third party or object. The flight response was exhibited by ignoring or avoiding the patient.

These types of reactions to difficult clients influence ethical decision making. Staff members should be encouraged to express such feelings and examine the conflict between their obligation to help clients and the client's right to self-determination. By discussing their feelings and understanding the values that underlie their actions, staff members can change the emotional context of the conflict and approach a resolution more rationally.

Reviewing the Case

This brief analysis of the ethical principles that underlie the case of Jane Langely does not provide one clear course of action for the home care agency involved in her care. However, this type of reflection helps to "clarify the moral problems created by the case and underline the considerations relevant to making a decision" (Jameton, 1983, p. 135).

Experienced home care providers may have read the case study with a jaundiced eye and wondered why Jane was discharged in the first place. In other words, they would not have taken the case under the circumstances presented. This view ends the discussion but provides no assistance to those home care providers involved in cases like Jane's.

To review the case, Jane appears to be a competent adult who is refusing to comply with her treatment regimen. Her refusal to comply in certain areas could result in life-threatening complications at worst and health-threatening complications at best. The attending physician, Dr. Abraham, has placed unrealistic, though commonly held, expectations on Jane, her family, and the home care agency regarding the time frame for twenty-four-hour skilled care. The home care agency will have to renegotiate this portion of their service agreement if Jane and her family want to continue care in the home.

Time is a positive factor in this case. After extending coverage beyond the thirty-day limit for twenty-four-hour skilled care, the home care provider needs to work with Jane and her parents regarding their expectations of home care. There is time to persuade Jane to change her mind. There is time for everyone involved to adjust to home care. There is time to explore other ways for Jane to assert her independence that are not as harmful.

The home care provider should examine its role in protecting Jane's privacy. The nurses on the case can work with Jane to set aside blocks of time during each shift so that Jane can be truly alone and yet safe. This would relieve some of the pressures caused by constant observation.

At this point, the risks do not appear high enough to withdraw from the case. However, the home care agency needs to be clear about where they will draw the line regarding the standard of Jane's care. There is a point at which care (or the lack of it) becomes dangerous and the home care agency can justifiably withdraw. Nurses and others who work with Jane may become concerned about their complicity in wrongdoing or harm. In other words, they may question their personal responsibility for Jane's welfare when she refuses to cooperate with the standards of basic, safe care. "One's responsibility grows as one becomes more closely involved in causing the harm" (Jameton, 1983, p. 130). The legal and moral issues of abandonment are discussed in greater detail in Chapter 9.

Thus, the home care agency must work with the field staff to decide what the safe standard of care will be in Jane's case so that no one feels he or she is participating in unsafe or harmful practices.

Once the standard is set and communicated to all those involved, including Jane and her parents, the home care provider must follow through with the standard or withdraw when it is not met.

The home care agency might also consider the use of a contract with Jane.

> A contract has been described as a vehicle for reducing conflict with "problem patients"—a strategy for defining and negotiating differences. The contract can maximize his sense of self-control and self-determination, qualities essential to long-term treatment and healing. (Quill, 1985, p. 16)

The home care agency can explore Jane's beliefs and requests and use them to establish a care plan with which both parties can live.

SUMMARY

A complex, high-tech home care case has been used to highlight key ethical principles central to caring for clients and their families. Conflicts between rights and responsibilities are common ethical problems in health care. Operational definitions of rights, responsibilities, and values have been provided in light of the case study. The client, Jane, is a young adult with a past history of strong independence now placed in a position of dependency on a ventilator, her parents, and her caregivers. Her parents are faced with the burden of caring for an adult-child. Their rights and responsibilities regarding her presence in their home is another source of ethical conflict. The home care providers' perspective includes their expectations of the client regarding self-care and compliance with treatment.

Focusing on the principal players in this case and their values, rights, and responsibilities helps sort out the ethical issues from other extraneous issues. The primary ethical principles that shape the home care provider–client relationship are autonomy and beneficence. The doctrine of informed consent was discussed in the context of home care, which differs in substance from the acute care setting. Various facets of the concept of autonomy were examined including the necessary conditions for an autonomous action and the problem of reduced autonomy.

Central to the principle of autonomy is the attitude of respectfulness toward the client. Respect for the client's decisions may run counter to the home care providers' obligation to do good for the client. These two principles are weighed in the balance when they conflict to determine the extent of the client's freedom and the home care providers' obligations.

The majority of home care providers will not have the time or the inclination to analyze a case this intensely. However, an appreciation of underlying values, rights, and responsibilities and an understanding of basic ethical principles provide the tools to analyze the ethical issues inherent in client care, to arrive at ethical choices in a rational manner, and to choose the best course of action.

REFERENCES

Allen, M. (1974). Ethics of nursing practice. *Canadian Nurse, 2*:22–24.

Beauchamp, T. (1986, June). *Autonomy.* Paper presented at the Kennedy Institute of Ethics, Intensive Bioethics Course, Washington, DC.

Beauchamp, T., & Childress, J. (1983). *Principles of Biomedical Ethics* (2nd ed.). New York: Oxford University Press.

Beauchamp, T., & Walters, L. (1982). *Contemporary Issues in Bioethics* (2nd ed.). Belmont, Calif: Wadsworth Publishing Company.

Carper, B.A. (1986). The ethics of caring. In P. Chinn (Ed.), *Ethical Issues in Nursing* (pp. 1–9). Rockville, Md: Aspen Systems Corp.

Childress, J. (1982). *Who Should Decide? Paternalism in Health Care.* New York: Oxford University Press.

Cohen, E.S. (1985). Autonomy and paternalism: Two goals in conflict. *Law, Medicine, and Health Care, 13*(4):145–150.

Cohen, C.B. (1987). Patient autonomy in chronic illness. *Family and Community Health, 10*(1):24–34.

Collopy, B. (1988). Autonomy in long term care: Some crucial distinctions. *The Gerontologist, 28*(Supplement):10–17.

Conrad, P. (1987). The noncompliant patient in search of autonomy. *The Hastings Center Report, 17*(4):15–17.

Dennis, K.E. (1987). Dimensions of client control. *Nursing Research, 36*:151–156.

Dudley, D.L., Glaser, E.M., Jorgenson, B.N., & Logan, D.L. (1980). Psychosocial concomitants to rehabilitation in chronic obstructive pulmonary disease: I. Psychosocial and psychological considerations. *Chest, 77*(3):413–420.

Dworkin, G. (1981). Taking risks, assessing responsibility. *Hastings Center Report, 11*(5):26–31.

Faden, R.R., & Beauchamp, T. (1987). *A History and Theory of Informed Consent.* New York: Oxford University Press.

Fromer, M.J. (1981). Paternalism in health care. *Nursing Outlook, 29*:284–290.

Haddad, A. (1987). *High Tech Home Care.* Rockville, Md: Aspen Publishers.

Highley, B., & Norris, C. (1957). When a student dislikes a patient. *American Journal of Nursing, 57*:1163–1166.

Jackson, D.L., & Youngner, S. (1979). Patient autonomy and 'death with dignity': Some clinical caveats. *The New England Journal of Medicine, 301*:404–408.

Jameton, A. (1983). Making hard choices. In S. Gorovitz, R. Macklin, A. Jameton, J.M. O'Connor, & S. Sherwin (Eds.), *Moral Problems in Medicine* (pp. 126–137). Englewood Cliffs, NJ: Prentice–Hall, Inc.

Jameton, A. (1988). In the borderlands of autonomy: Responsibility in long term care facilities. *The Gerontologist, 28*(Supplement):18–23.
Jonsen, A.R., Siegler, M., & Winslade, W.J. (1982). *Clinical Ethics.* New York: Macmillan Publishing Company.
Keller, N.S. (1971). Compliance, previous access and provision of services by registered nurses. *Journal of Health and Social Behavior, 12*: 321–330.
Kelly, M., & May, D. (1982). Good and bad patients: A review of the literature and a theoretical critique. *Journal of Advanced Nursing, 7*:147–156.
Kravitz, M. (1985). Informed consent: Must ethical responsibility conflict with professional conduct? *Nursing Management, 16*(11):34A–34H.
Lambert, C., & Lambert, V. (1987). Psychosocial impacts created by chronic illness. *Nursing Clinics of North America, 22*:527–533.
Mattsson, E.I. (1975). Psychological aspects of severe physical injury and its treatment. *The Journal of Trauma, 15*:217–233.
Miller, B. (1981). Autonomy and the refusal of lifesaving treatment. *Hastings Center Report, 11*(4):22–28.
Parsons, T. (1951). *The Social System.* Glencoe, Ill: The Free Press.
Podrasky, D.L., & Sexton, D. (1988). Nurses' reactions to difficult patients. *Image, 20*(1):16–21.
Post, S. (1987). Family ethics in caring for newborns with impairments. *Health Progress, 68*(5):57–61.
Power, P.W. (1989). Working with families: An intervention model for rehabilitation nurses. *Rehabilitation Nursing, 14*(2):73–76.
President's Commission for the Study of Ethical Problems in Medicine and Biomedical and Behavioral Research. (1983). *Summing Up.* Washington, DC: US Government Printing Office.
Quill, T. (1985). Patient centered medicine: Increasing patient responsibility. *Hospital Practice, 20*(11A):6–17.
Salladay, S., & Haddad, A. (1986). Point-counterpoint technique in assessing hidden agendas. *Dimensions in Critical Care, 5*:238–243.
Siegler, M. (1977). Critical illness: The limits of autonomy. *Hastings Center Report, 7*(5):12–15.
Stuifbergen, A.K. (1987). The impact of chronic illness on families. *Family and Community Health, 9*(4):43–51.
Tagliaczzo, D.L., & Mauksch, H.O. (1979). The patient's view of the patient's role. In E.G. Jaco (Ed.), *Patients, Physicians and Illness* (3rd ed.). New York: Macmillan Publishing Company.
Tisdale, S. (1986). *The Sorcerer's Apprentice.* New York: Harper & Row.
Watson, P.G. (1987). Family participation in the rehabilitation process: The rehabilitator's perspective. *Rehabilitation Nursing, 12*(2):70–73.
Youngner, S. (1986). Patient autonomy, informed consent, and the reality of critical care. *Critical Care Clinics, 2*(1):41–52.
Zaner, R.M. (1974). The unanchored leaf: Humanities and the discipline of care. *Texas Reports on Biology and Medicine, 32*(1):1–18.

Chapter 4

Withholding and Withdrawing Treatment

Amy Marie Haddad
Marshall B. Kapp

Decisions by clients, families, and health care professionals not to intervene medically in the natural process of dying have occurred for years. Perhaps these decisions were easier to make in the past as medical science had limited ability to alter the course of the disease process and the dying trajectory. Medical technology has changed dramatically, however, and the ability to prolong life for long periods of time through advanced cardiopulmonary and nutritional support is a clinical fact. This includes individuals in irreversible comas, those who are imminently going to die, or those in a persistent vegetative state. Families and health care professionals anguish over what is best for the client, whether treatments such as ventilators, feeding tubes, and total parenteral nutrition are helpful or harmful, and most basically, when enough is enough.

For most people, the goal of medical care—and home care—is not, and has not been, the maintenance of life at all costs. It is important, therefore, that home care providers develop guidelines that ensure that medical treatment does not become an absolute and that the client is treated with dignity. This chapter explains some of the major ethical debates and legal decisions that have surrounded the complex issue of life-sustaining treatments.

ETHICAL ASPECTS

According to the report of the President's Commission for the Study of Ethical Problems in Medicine and Biomedical and Behavioral Research (1983), the hallmark of ethically sound decision making in health care in general and about life-sustaining treatments in particular is that it enables competent and informed clients to reach voluntary decisions about their care. The right to make decisions about medical care includes the right to refuse treatment. This right receives its ethical justification from the principle of autonomy (see Chapter 3). Autonomy is the basis for informed consent as well as the right to refuse care. The right to refuse treatment is not absolute, but countervailing interests must be substantial to outweigh the wishes of a competent client.

Additional ethical principles that are helpful in analyzing the issue of withholding and withdrawing treatment are beneficence and nonmaleficence. Nonmaleficence is sometimes viewed as a subset of the principle of beneficence. But in the case of withdrawing life-sustaining treatment, it is helpful to view nonmaleficence as a distinct principle. Nonmaleficence requires that we not harm others, which obviously includes not killing. Thus, deliberately engaging in actions that bring about, hasten, or cause death is an obvious wrong as a violation of the principle of nonmaleficence (United States Office of Technology Assessment, 1987). Killing is generally forbidden except in the cases of self-defense, war, and capital punishment. Most ethical traditions hold this principle to be of primary importance and therefore prohibit the direct killing of innocent persons even if they are suffering greatly.

In examining the mandate to avoid harm, it is important to look beyond the mere physical aspect of the individual in question. A person, for example, is more than a cardiopulmonary system, a gastrointestinal system, a mind, and more, and cannot be really understood by looking at these parts alone. Each person has various dimensions that must be integrated to avoid harming the client.

> One aspect of the person is the physiological; the person's physical aspects must be seen as central since no person exists outside of a body. This concern is not necessarily the most important aspect of the person, since a person's body exists to help that person attain or pursue other values—spiritual, social, familial, and so on. As a result, maintaining the physical part of human life is an important value and responsibility, but not necessarily the ultimate value. (O'Rourke & Brodeur, 1989, p. 189)

Other principles that figure prominently in the discussion of withholding and withdrawing treatment are justice, fidelity, and veracity (see Chapter 1).

DISTINCTIONS REGARDING LIFE-SUSTAINING TREATMENT

In decisions about life-sustaining treatment, numerous terms are used and often inappropriately applied. Because of this, discussions regarding withholding or withdrawing treatment can be confusing and anxiety provoking. What does it mean to use "aggressive treatment?" What does "no heroic measures" mean? Is it the same as "do not resuscitate?" It is essential that those involved in decisions about life-sustaining treatment speak the same language. The following discussion will examine distinctions between the most commonly used terms and clarify their various meanings and their application to home care practice.

Foregoing Treatment

To forego life-sustaining treatment means to do without a medical intervention that would be expected to extend the client's life. Foregoing includes both the noninitiation of treatment and the discontinuance of an ongoing treatment. The term "forego" encompasses both withholding and withdrawing treatment.

Withholding versus Withdrawing

Some hold that there is no moral difference between withholding treatment that would be essentially futile or withdrawing care after it has been initiated (President's Commission, 1983). Many health care providers feel that there is a clear distinction between withholding and withdrawing treatment, based largely on the principle of fidelity. The relationship between health care provider and client implies certain promises. The promise of "doing good" for the client is implicit. This doing good involves treating and caring for the client. Some health care professionals have been trained to do everything possible to support life. However, there is no promise to continue futile treatment. For psychological reasons, not moral or legal ones, withdrawing treatment is more difficult than withholding treatment.

The following case illustrates the distinction between withholding and withdrawing treatment.

Case 4–1. Discontinuing Treatment

Chloe was born with trisomy 18, an abnormal chromosome count that resulted in multiple congenital malformations, including those of the ears, hands, gastrointestinal tract, and heart. Chloe had spent the two first months of her life in the neonatal intensive care unit. Chloe was not a candidate for cardiac surgery and without the surgery was not likely to survive more than a few months. Chloe's parents decided to take her home with the understanding that she would be a "no code" (no attempts to initiate cardiopulmonary resuscitation) in the event of a cardiac or respiratory arrest. The home care provider on the case was comfortable with this decision as it could be viewed as withholding treatment that would not be beneficial to Chloe and only prevent her imminent death.

Chloe continued to receive gastrostomy feedings, intermittent suctioning through her tracheostomy, and several cardiovascular drugs from her home care nurses. During a care conference with Chloe's pediatrician, Dr. Lazer, some of the nurses questioned continuing the use of medications such as atropine and furosemide. Others on the team felt strongly that the medications should be continued along with measures to keep her airway clear and provide nutrition. Those who wanted to continue to provide her with nutrition argued that, "We owe her that much at least—to support her until it is no longer effective. After all, we are talking about feeding her, not any sophisticated treatment."

Chloe's parents' decision to make her a "no code" is an example of withholding a specific treatment—cardiopulmonary resuscitation. The staff's discussion regarding the discontinuation of Chloe's cardiovascular drugs involves withdrawing treatment. The staff's reluctance to remove support they are already providing is obvious.

In addition to the principle of fidelity, there is the emotional bond that ties the home care provider and the client together which makes it difficult to withdraw care. The closer we get to clients, the harder it is to let go. Therefore, some health care providers are reluctant to start treatments in order to avoid the trauma of withdrawing them later. "Yet, it is often necessary to start life-sustaining treatments to gain time and information for better diagnosis, prognosis, and decision making" (United States Office of Technology Assessment, 1987). In other words, by trying a specific treatment we can eliminate some of the clinical ambiguity common to these types of cases and more accurately gauge the benefit or futility of the treatment. This provides a more solid foundation for removing or discontinuing treatment than if it had never been tried.

Direct versus Indirect

The distinction between direct and indirect actions has traditionally rested on the principle of double effect. This principle supports the claim that some actions that produce a harmful effect, such as death, are not always morally prohibited. The application of the principle of double effect is illustrated in the following case:

Case 4–2. Pain Management in Terminal Illness

Marge George, a 54-year-old woman, is in the terminal stages of metastatic cancer of the breast. Marge has received every type of traditional treatment and therapy available but to no avail. Marge wants to return home. The clinical supervisor from the home care agency the Georges have selected meets with Marge's physician, Dr. Foster, to discuss the plan of care. Dr. Foster states that Marge needs supportive care and pain management. Dr. Foster orders an ambulatory infusion pump to deliver a continuous dose of morphine, which can be supplemented by boluses of morphine if necessary.

As the disease progresses, Marge becomes weaker and requires higher and higher doses of morphine to relieve her pain. The nurse on the case realizes that increasing the dose of morphine will eventually cause respiratory depression and subsequent death, yet Marge had made it clear from the outset that she did not want to suffer unnecessarily.

The Principle of Double Effect. The principle of double effect involves four conditions that are evident in Marge's case: (1) The action in itself must be good or at least morally neutral. The action in question is pain management, which is in itself good. (2) The person intending the action (in this case, the nurse) must intend only the good effect and not the evil effect. The evil effect is foreseen but not intended. The good effect is relief of Marge's pain. The evil effect is respiratory depression, which will result in Marge's eventual death. The nurse intends only the good effect, to relieve Marge's pain, not Marge's death even though it is foreseen. (3) The evil effect cannot be a means to the good effect. That is, the good and evil effects must follow immediately from the same action (Beauchamp & Childress, 1983). (4) There must be proportionality between the good and the evil effects for the action; that is, there must be a proportionally stronger reason for allowing the evil effect to occur. In Marge's case, the good that is brought about by pain relief in a terminally ill person outweighs the unintended evil effect of eventual death.

Killing and Letting Die

For many people, the term "killing" is always wrong and "letting die" can sometimes be morally correct. The use of these terms is often confusing and other distinctions have been used such as: commission and omission, and active and passive euthanasia. Regardless of the words, the distinction between these terms

> . . . does not necessarily determine moral conclusions about particular cases. For instance, it is possible to reject the distinction and to hold that some cases of what have been called "killing" and "letting die" are morally permissible, or that all cases are morally prohibited; and it is also possible to affirm the distinction and yet hold that most cases of letting die and all cases of killing are morally wrong. (Beauchamp & Childress, 1983, pp. 116–117).

The ethical issues remain, however, and the home care provider must be able to draw a line between the two concepts. As mentioned previously, most ethical traditions prohibit active killing. The most common argument for active killing is to relieve intractable pain and suffering on the part of a dying client. This is most often referred to as "mercy killing." The motivation for mercy killing is not malice but sympathy, compassion, and a desire to help the client out of an unbearable situation. However, in mercy killing cases, sympathy and compassion are not considered adequate provocation. The legal prohibition against active, direct killing is quite clear.

In addition to the legal prohibitions, there are several arguments that oppose mercy killing on other grounds. First of all, there are numerous, effective, and often untried measures that can relieve a client's pain. Secondly, the possibility for abuse is high. People might hasten the deaths of family members in order to avoid the burden of caregiving or suffering through the dying process that is often unpredictable and emotionally draining. There do not appear to be sufficient reasons to change the prohibition against active killing.

The American Medical Association's Council on Ethical and Judicial Affairs has determined that for humane reasons, with informed consent, a physician may do what is medically necessary to alleviate severe pain or cease or omit treatment to permit a terminally ill client whose death is imminent to die. However, the physician should not intentionally cause death (Council on Ethical and Judicial Affairs, 1986). Letting die involves the withholding or termination of treatment in cases where the possibility for extending life under humane and comfortable conditions is extremely small. This may involve the withholding of certain medications, such as antibiotics, or the removal of ventilator support, or the withdrawal of nutrition and hydration. Of course, none of these actions can be considered without the consent of the client or, when that is not possible, the consent of a legally valid surrogate.

The distinction between killing and letting die is particularly important in the context of home care. In an institutional setting, there are numerous individuals involved in client care, which decreases the chance for illegal activities such as active killing, abuse, and neglect. Institutions are open to the public. The possibility of hidden "mercy killings" in home care is high. "It will be very difficult to monitor what goes on behind those millions of closed doors" (Bayer, 1986). Since monitoring will be difficult, each home care provider must be clear about the legal and moral prohibitions against killing and the justifications for letting die.

Ordinary and Extraordinary Means

The distinction between "ordinary" and "extraordinary" means of treatment, originally formulated in Roman Catholic theology, has a long history in medical treatment decisions. Ordinary treatment is required and extraordinary treatment is not required. That is, an individual can refuse extraordinary treatment and the action not labeled as suicide. But what is extraordinary treatment?

Once again, there is considerable confusion about what the two terms mean. Ordinary treatment is often wrongly taken to mean usual, customary, inexpensive, and available, whereas extraordinary treatment is conversely viewed as unusual and expensive. These interpretations focus on the properties of medical practice rather than the efficacy of the treatment in question and the burden of treatment as interpreted by the client.

One interpretation of the distinction embodies the following criteria: for a therapy to be obligatory it must offer a reasonable hope of benefit and not involve excessive expense, pain, or other inconvenience (Kelly, 1951). The reference to proportionate benefits and burdens of treatment as viewed by particular clients is advocated. Therefore, any medical treatment—including hydration, antibiotics, transfusions, cardiopulmonary resuscitation—could be construed as "extraordinary" and not obligatory if it is out of proportion with the client's interests and wishes or holds little hope of benefit.

Finally, an understanding of the client's physical condition is necessary for an understanding of treatment decisions. In addition to the ethical framework, four medical criteria should be carefully examined when determining whether to discontinue life-sustaining treatment, especially in cases of irreversible coma or persistent vegetative state: (1) the accuracy of the diagnosis; (2) the certainty of the prognosis; (3) the options for treatment; and (4) the probable consequences of non-treatment (Miller, 1988).

THE ETHICS OF WITHDRAWING FEEDING AND HYDRATION

All the ethical distinctions presented for withholding and withdrawing treatment allow clients or their surrogate decision makers to determine whether the probable benefit of treatment outweighs its probable burdens from the client's perspective and to refuse any treatment. There has been considerable debate about whether this also includes artificial sustenance. Food and fluids have been treated as unique forms of treatment by some. The rationale for this includes the following:

1. The denial of food and fluids is distinguishable from denial of medical and surgical therapy in one respect, which may be called "finality." The denial of food and fluids is biologically final in a way, and with a degree of certainty, that the denial of other therapy is not (Derr, 1986).
2. Food and fluids may be necessary for comfort and dignity.
3. Food and fluids symbolize care and compassion on the most basic level, and their withdrawal from vulnerable individuals signifies a threat to the foundation of humane care (Callahan, 1983).

Others have argued that artificially supplied food and fluids should be treated the same as any other medical treatment in that if it offers no substantial hope of benefit to the client, he has no moral obligation to undergo it, nor the physician to order it (Paris, 1986). The necessity for food and fluids as a comfort measure has been countered with the following arguments:

> First, dying by withdrawal of food and fluid, or by withdrawal of a respirator, is not usually and need never be uncomfortable for the dying person. Although very little is published on the subject, physicians and nurses who care for dying persons without artificial feeding are hard pressed to recall patients who evidenced or voiced hunger or thirst, even with striking objective evidence of dehydration, starvation ketosis, and weight loss (historical accounts of death from chronic disease before modern tubes also do not mention patients suffering from starvation or thirst). (Lynn, 1984)

Withdrawal of medical treatment never includes the withdrawal of nursing care and support for the client. Sensitive, supportive care of clients from whom medical treatment has been withheld or withdrawn is of primary importance.

MAKING THE DECISION

Important procedural questions center around who decides if and when treatment is to be discontinued. Client mental capacity is central to the determination of the client's wishes (past and present) regarding treatment decisions. This will be examined in greater detail in the following section on the legal aspects of withholding and withdrawing treatment.

Regardless of who makes the decision, it is important to examine the ethics and process of decision making. The home care provider cannot expect a client (or family member) to make up his or her mind to forego treatment in a single session. As the client's condition and options, not to mention understanding and evaluations, are far from static, discussions must continue throughout the delivery of home care services (Nolan, 1987). However, the home care provider should not avoid the discussion. The practice of waiting until an emergency situation to decide to forego treatment is procedurally and ethically inferior to advance planning.

There is a need for ongoing, open discussions with the client and family. Language should be as clear and unambiguous as possible. Treatment options should be spelled out in lay terms. Family members may not know how to or be afraid to ask certain questions. Therefore, if there are no questions this does not necessarily mean that the family or client fully understands the options that have been presented to them.

The consequences of the various treatment options should also be explored. For example, if the client has made the decision to forego cardiopulmonary resuscitation and will likely progress into pulmonary edema, the family should be warned of this possibility. This might include a description of anticipated changes in breathing, level of consciousness, and the client's color. Many lay people have a romantic notion of what "death with dignity" means and are completely unprepared for the reality of a death in the home. The home care provider must use sensitive timing to present this sort of information to the family. Though these discussions require a great deal of courage, they offer the opportunity to clarify treatment goals, acknowledge the gravity of the prognosis, and realistically deal with the dying process.

LEGAL ASPECTS

Almost all of the legal cases presenting issues of withholding or withdrawing life-sustaining medical treatment that have arisen thus far have occurred within the context of institutional—that is, acute care hospital or nursing home—settings (Meisel, 1989). However, this phenomenon is likely to change significantly in the coming years. Because "[many] people wish to die at home in familiar surroundings [a]nd, in many cases, hospitals discharge terminally or irreversibly ill patients. . .medical care in the home, especially for terminally and irreversibly ill patients, is increasing" (*In re Farrell*, 1987).

As technologies such as dialysis, mechanical ventilation, antibiotic therapy, and artificial nutrition and hydration become more commonplace as a part of home care services for increasingly sicker clients (United States Office of Technology Assessment, 1987), decisions about the legal permissibility or propriety of limiting those treatments for some clients in particular circumstances will become more and more perplexing for home care providers. While every situation is influenced by its own specific facts, home care providers should be guided in this difficult area of decision making by several legal principles that are emerging as legislatures and the courts grapple with these issues. Although most of the legal precedent to date has been forged in the environment of institutional health care, as a matter of logic and policy these emerging legal principles ought to be applied with full force to guide medical decision making in the client's home.

COMPETENT CLIENTS

As noted in Chapter 3, an essential element of legally and ethically effective medical decision making (along with voluntariness and a sufficient amount of information) is the presence of a mentally capable decision maker. This requirement applies whether a particular medical intervention is being consented to or declined, and whether the place for decision making is a health care institution or the client's home (O'Neil, 1987).

Thus, the threshold question in arriving at any medical decision, including decisions to limit life-sustaining interventions, is whether the client has adequate mental capacity (in legal phraseology, in most states, "competency") to make treatment decisions for him- or herself. Definitions of decision-making competency are a matter of individual state law, with most states defining competency in a very unclear and imprecise manner. A thorough discussion of the concept of legal competence is beyond the scope of this chapter (see generally Haddad, 1988; Kapp, 1987, chap. 6; Kapp, 1988, chap. 2, Kapp & Bigot, 1985, chaps. 3 & 8), but a few basic points should be noted.

First, every adult (in virtually every state, in the medical decision making realm this refers to people older than 18) is legally presumed to be competent to make his or her own medical decisions. The burden of proof rests with those who are claiming that a client lacks decision making capacity. Technically, the presumption of competence can be overcome and a substitute decision maker (see next section) appointed only upon a decision by a state probate court that the client lacks the minimum functional capacity to engage in a rational thinking process concerning the particular decision confronting the client and its consequences. A competence determination centers on the client's functioning, and not merely the client's clinical diagnosis.

Second, the legislatures and courts have held uniformly that a mentally competent individual has a fundamental right to make his or her own medical decisions. This right is based on the constitutional right to privacy, the common-law right of bodily integrity, and the constitutional right to free exercise of religion.

Government may override the competent individual's right to choose, even if that choice is exercised to decline life-sustaining treatment, only in those very rare instances where government (society) has a compelling interest in doing so. For instance, a client who can probably be restored to normal, productive functioning as a result of a relatively short period of medical intervention, who has a dire prognosis without intervention, and who is the parent of minor children who need support might be forced by a court to receive such medical intervention in order to further society's compelling interest in protecting innocent third parties. Conversely, in most home care situations, where the client does not have dependent minor children and is not likely to return to any semblance of normal, productive capacity as a consequence of medical intervention, there is no compelling government interest to justify overriding the competent client's right to choose his or her own destiny. Hence, the very strong weight of legal opinion, in most home care situations, would command respect for the competent patient's limitation-of-treatment wishes.

In the major home care legal decision concerning a competent client, 37-year-old Kathleen Farrell, (*In re Farrell*, 1987) was diagnosed as having amyotrophic lateral sclerosis, or "Lou Gehrig's disease." She had been on a respirator at home for three years and wanted to have the machine disconnected. Her husband, two teen-age sons, and physician all agreed to her request. The husband petitioned the New Jersey trial level court for permission to exercise his competent wife's choice to have the respirator removed. After visiting Mrs. Farrell in her home, the judge found her competent and authorized her husband to comply with her wishes.

On appeal (brought by Mrs. Farrell's *guardian ad litem* appointed by the court), the New Jersey Supreme Court affirmed Mrs. Farrell's right as a competent home care client to make choices—even regarding the limitation of life-sustaining treatment—about her own medical destiny. This decision set out some guidelines for the determination of a client's decision making capacity. This determination, according to the *Farrell* opinion, is to be made by the attending physician and confirmed by two other physicians. There need not be a judicial determination of competence, in part because clients are legally presumed to be competent and in part because of the requirement for independent confirmation. The attending physician must provide the client with information adequate to permit the client to render an informed consent about foregoing life-sustaining treatment and must also ensure that the client's decision is a voluntary, uncoerced one. The two independent physicians must also confirm that the client's decision is voluntary and informed. Not surprisingly, the court was silent on the issue of who pays for the services of the two confirming physicians.

Voluntary industry standards are to the same effect in terms of emphasis on the decision making autonomy of the competent client. When a client is not personally functionally capable of engaging in a rational decision making process, someone else must act as a substitute (sometimes called a surrogate or proxy) to exercise the client's rights on the client's behalf. This includes the client's right to accept or reject medical intervention.

SUBSTITUTE DECISION MAKERS

When a client is not personally functionally capable of engaging in a rational decision making process, someone else must act as a substitute (sometimes called a surrogate or proxy) to exercise the client's rights on the client's behalf. This includes the client's right to accept or reject medical intervention.

Delegating Decisional Authority

The transfer of decision making authority from a client to a substitute may occur in a variety of ways. The client, while still competent, may write out a document such as a *durable power of attorney* that delegates authority to another named person upon the happening of a specified event (such as the client's incompetence as verified by a physician). In a growing number of states (approximately a dozen as of this time), legislatures are enacting *family consent statutes* that empower specified family members to make medical decisions for incompetent clients where the client while still competent expressed no preference to the contrary (Areen, 1987). Home care agencies must be familiar with their own state statutes on durable power of attorney and family consent.

Guardianship

The most common legal mechanism for substitute medical decision making is *guardianship of the person* (in some states, like California, called *conservatorship).* Guardianship is a legal relationship established by a state probate court where it finds that a person (the ward) is not capable of making his or her own decisions and it appoints another person (the guardian) to make decisions for the ward. Traditionally, the guardian has been expected to make decisions that are in the ward's *best interests*, but recently courts and legislatures have been moving toward a *substituted judgment* standard. Under substituted judgment, the guardian is expected to make decisions consistent with the personal values and preferences of the ward, that is, to try as well as possible to approximate those decisions that the ward would make personally if currently able to engage in a rational decision making process. Courts have differed over the degree of proof required to establish what the incompetent individual would have wanted done in particular circumstances.

Because the guardianship mechanism often has been misused in the past to deprive persons of fundamental decisional rights unnecessarily, there is substantial activity in state legislatures today aimed at limiting the appointment and powers of guardians (Parry, 1988). With increasing frequency the powers delegated to guardians by the probate courts are less than total (total guardianship over all personal and property decisions usually being referred to as *plenary*). It is important for home care agencies, when dealing with family members or others who claim to have guardianship authority concerning a client, to verify both the existence and the extent of that authority. The agency should insist on being provided with any relevant court documents appointing the substitute, should read such documents carefully, refer any questions to the agency's attorney (see Chapter 8), and should place a copy of such documents in the client's medical record maintained by the agency.

Clients Without Advance Directives or Guardians

Where the client has not (or because of lifelong disability could not have) prepared for eventual incapacity through an advance planning document such as a durable power of attorney, one's jurisdiction does not have a family consent statute in effect, and no formal guardianship proceeding has been initiated for a specific client, a further mechanism of substitute decision making is possible. This is the process of informal, extralegal decision making that occurs ubiquitously within the health care system, in institutional and community-based settings, every day. There are a sizable number of clients in hospitals, nursing homes, and certainly in home care settings, who are *de facto* but not *de jure* incompetent, that is, who in fact lack the capacity to engage in a rational decision making process concerning their own medical futures by themselves, but who have not been formally declared incompetent by a court. For such persons, initiating the expensive, time-consuming, and emotionally draining process of guardianship, although that process is the only available way to absolutely delineate the formal legal rights and responsibilities of all parties, seems foolish where family members or close friends who are truly acting in the client's best interests are involved.

Acting on the basis of informed but informal discussion and agreement among concerned family or friends, the physician, and other members of the health care team, including home care agency administration, exposes the agency and its staff to very slight legal risk, even where the decision is to limit life-sustaining medical treatment for a client who no longer can benefit from such treatment. Of course, where legal warning signals are apparent (eg, serious and irreconcilable disagreement among family members or between the family and the health care team, or family members making decisions contrary to the clear best interests or known personal preferences of the client), the home care agency should consult its legal counsel and consider requesting the family to initiate a formal guardianship action.

ADVANCE DIRECTIVES

Through available legal mechanisms of advance planning, a person may take steps while still mentally capable to anticipate and prepare for eventual incapacity by directing future medical treatment or voluntarily delegating future medical decision making power. At present, there are two primary mechanisms for advance health care planning.

Living Wills

A *living will* is a document that allows a person to give specific advance directions concerning medical treatment in the event of subsequent mental incapacity. As of 1989, forty states plus the District of Columbia (see Appendix 4A) had enacted statutes specifically authorizing the execution of a living will (or "natural death") document. In addition, courts in several states without living will statutes have ruled that the written directive of a competent person concerning future medical treatment is entitled to be given legal standing after the person becomes incompetent. Living will statutes vary in detail from state to state. In addition to providing a mechanism for expressing future treatment preferences, the living will under many state statutes may also be used by people to designate another individual as their representative and substitute decision maker in the event of future incapacity.

Durable Power of Attorney For Health Care

The *durable power of attorney* (discussed earlier) is a legal document in which an individual (the *principal*) may direct, through the appointment of an *agent* (the "attorney-in-fact," who need not be an attorney-at-law) the making of medical decisions in the event of future incapacity. The principal may give the agent general or specific instructions to direct future decision making. Every state has a durable power of attorney statute. This device traditionally has been used mainly for asset management purposes. In the last few years, several states have enacted statutes explicitly creating a *durable power of attorney for health care*. Even in states without such specific statutes, there appears to be no reason to prevent the general durable power of attorney statute from applying to medical decisions.

Durable powers of attorney fall into two categories. An *immediate* power comes into effect immediately upon the naming of an agent. In a *springing* power, the legal authority is transferred ("springs") from the principal to the agent only upon the occurrence of some specified future event, such as confirmation of the principal's incapacity by an examining physician.

Home care agencies must have written policies and procedures for determining whether a client has executed a living will or durable power of attorney. The home care agency must develop and maintain a close working relationship with the substitute decision maker, if any, to whom a client has delegated decision making authority. The home care agency should obtain a copy of any purported advance planning document executed by a client, should verify the document's authenticity, and should place that copy of the document in the client's permanent file. The agency must also have written policies and procedures for communicating a client's advance directive status to relevant staff, in a manner that is effective in ensuring that the client's wishes are respected but that also protects the client's right to confidentiality.

"DO NOT" ORDERS

"Do not" orders may be written by the client's physician (and only by the physician). These orders are predicated on prospectively made decisions—ideally resulting from full discussion between the physician, other members of the health care team, and the client or client's substitute decision maker—to withdraw or withhold certain types of medical interventions from specified clients. Most attention thus far has been devoted to "do not resuscitate" (DNR) orders ("no codes"), or instructions by the physician to refrain from attempts at cardiopulmonary resuscitation in the event of a cardiac arrest. However, other kinds of "do not" orders also are important, especially in the home care environment, such as "do not hospitalize" and "do not treat" orders.

Legally, "do not" orders should be handled according to the same substantive principles and procedural guidelines that apply to other treatment decisions (*Matter of Dinnerstein*, 1978). By allowing and encouraging certain decisions to be made *prospectively*, before a crisis develops, "do not" orders may reduce potential legal risk and should curtail legal anxiety.

A *competent* adult client has the right voluntarily to refuse basic or advance cardiac life support or any of its specific components, or any other form of medical intervention including hospitalization, and to demand that he or she be the recipient of a precisely written "do not" order.

For the *mentally incompetent* client, clarification of respective rights and responsibilities may be available from the client's previously executed directive or from discussions with an authorized proxy. In the absence of such clarification, "do not" orders are still permissible for incompetent clients according to the same general legal principles governing other kinds of decisions about life-sustaining medical treatment. This involves balancing, from the client's perspective, the reasonably foreseeable benefits and burdens of the particular medical intervention.

Before writing and implementing a "do not" order for an incompetent client with no advance directive or current legally appointed proxy, the physician should consult with any available family members or close friends of the client and with other members of the health care team, and should carefully document his or her orders and their underlying reasons. "Do not" orders should be subject to regular review for appropriateness; if the clinical condition of the client changes, a "do not" order should be rethought. In short, the only pertinent distinction between "do not" orders and other decisions to limit life-sustaining interventions lies in the prospective nature of the former.

Home care agencies should develop written policies and procedures regarding the entry of "do not" orders for clients. (As noted below, agencies are required by JCAHO standards to do this for DNR orders.) Provisions must be included regarding the decision making involvement of authorized substitute decision makers, family and friends without formal legal authorization but who function in practice as substitute decision makers, the competent client, and members of the health care team; checking for advance directives; documentation of "do not" orders and their underlying rationales; and communication of "do not" status to relevant home care staff. The agency's policies and procedures also must spell out the relationship of the home care agency and the client's attending physician concerning "do not" orders, expectations of the physician in this regard, and means of monitoring the physician's satisfaction of those expectations and of correcting communication or documentation problems. It should be emphasized that only a licensed physician—and not the home care agency acting independently—may enter a valid "do not" order. Agency staff should receive in-service training regarding the implementation of "do not" orders.

LEGAL ASPECTS OF ARTIFICIAL FEEDING AND HYDRATION

The most controversial issue today in the area of withholding and withdrawing life-sustaining treatment is how artificial means of nutrition and hydration ought to be characterized. Whether feeding and hydrating clients through tubes is viewed as a medical procedure or as a more basic, primordial form of nurturing will determine the legal propriety of withholding or withdrawing that intervention from a client.

This issue has been presented to the courts in a number of jurisdictions. The strong weight of legal authority emerging from cases that have raised this issue is that artificial feeding tubes should be categorized as a form of medical treatment, and therefore they may be subject to being withheld or withdrawn according to the same substantive and procedural principles as other medical treatments. It is important to note, however, that the highest court in at least one state (Missouri) recently has reached a contrary conclusion, holding that it is never legally permissible to limit artificial feeding that is prolonging an individual's life. In summary, the Missouri Supreme court stated,

> Given the fact that Nancy is alive and that the burdens of her treatment are not excessive for her, we do not believe her right to refuse treatment, whether that right proceeds from a constitutional right of privacy or a common law right to refuse treatment, outweighs the immense, clear fact of life in which the state maintains a vital interest. *(Cruzan v Harmon*, 1988)

As this chapter is written, the United States Supreme Court has this Missouri decision *(Cruzan v Director Missouri Department of Health*, 1989) under review, with an opinion due in 1990.

The issue is complicated by the fact that the living will statutes enacted in a number of states contain provisions that explicitly purport to prevent competent individuals from refusing in advance artificial means of nutrition and hydration (and implicitly or explicitly to prevent substitute decision makers from refusing artificial feeding for incompetent persons). These statutes, such as the one under review by the Supreme Court currently in *Cruzan*, specifically assert that nutrition and hydration, even if accomplished through tubes, are fundamentally different from medical treatments that may appropriately be withheld or withdrawn in certain circumstances. In the only case besides *Cruzan* thus far testing the validity of such a provision in a living will statute, a Florida District Court invalidated the provision on the grounds that a competent person possesses a constitutional and common-law right to refuse unwanted interventions—even feeding tubes—and that right takes precedence over legislation enacted by the state seeking to eliminate that right (*Corbett v D'Alessandro*, 1986). Even in Florida, the issue is being relitigated at the time of this writing in another case where a previously competent patient sought to guard against later artificial feeding (*Browning*, 1989). The validity of statutory provisions excluding the possibility of refusing artificial feeding mechanisms remains in question in those other states that have such a provision in their living will law but as yet no court decision interpreting it.

Home care agencies are advised to develop written policies and procedures regarding the withholding or withdrawing of artificial nutrition and hydration. These policies and procedures should be written in consultation with the agency's legal counsel, especially after review of the *Cruzan* case. It may also be wise to submit drafts of these policies and procedures to state licensing authorities and certifying agencies for their comments prior to formal adoption by the agency. These policies and procedures should deal with the agency's relationship with attending physicians, who are the only ones authorized by law to write orders to withhold or withdraw any form of life-sustaining interventions. Extensive in-service training on this issue is also necessary.

AGENCY POLICIES AND PROCEDURES

To reiterate a point made repeatedly throughout this chapter, home care agencies need to develop, in consultation with their legal counsels, written policies and procedures on the range of issues discussed here. JCAHO Standard HH.10 for Accreditation of Home Care requires that "The home care organization has written policies and procedures regarding the resuscitation of patients and for documentation in the home care record, including, as appropriate, provisions for appropriate orders by the patient's/client's physician." While resuscitation is a problem that already has received a great deal of legal and ethical attention, the other issues raised in this chapter should also be covered in agency policies and procedures.

SUMMARY

Careful policies and procedures, forged through a thoughtful and deliberative process and conscientiously implemented, can be valuable in assisting an agency to avoid legal and regulatory difficulties and to treat clients in a more humane and ethical manner (Miles & Gomez, 1989).

REFERENCES

Areen, J. (1987). The legal status of consent obtained from families of adult patients to withhold or withdraw treatment. *Journal of the American Medical Association, 258*:229–235.

Bayer, R. (1986). Ethics in home care and quality assurance. *Caring, 5*(1):50–56.

Beauchamp, T., & Childress, J.F. (1983). *Principles of Biomedical Ethics* (2nd ed.). New York: Oxford University Press.

Callahan, D. (1983). On feeding the dying. *Hastings Center Report, 13*(5):22.

Corbett v D'Alessandro, 487 So2d 368 (Fla Dist Ct App), *review denied*, 492 So2d 1331 (Fla 1986).

Council on Ethical and Judicial Affairs. (1986). Statement on withholding and withdrawing life prolonging medical treatment. *Journal of the American Medical Association, 256*:471.

Cruzan v Harmon, 760 SW2d 408, 416 (Mo 1988) (*en banc*).

Cruzan v Director of Missouri Department of Health, 760 SW2d 408 (1988), *cert granted*, No. 88-1503 (US Sup Ct).

Derr, P. (1986). Why food and fluids can never be denied. *Hastings Center Report, 16*(1):28–30.

Haddad, A.M. (1988). Determining competency. *Journal of Gerontological Nursing, 14*(6):19–22.

In the Guardianship of Browning, 543 So2d 258 (1989), on appeal to Florida Supreme Court.

In re Farrell, 108 NJ 335, 529 A2d 404 (1987).

Joint Commission on Accreditation of Healthcare Organizations. (1988). *1988 Home Care Standards for Accreditation*. Chicago: Joint Commission on Accreditation of Healthcare Organizations.

Kapp, M.B. (1987). *Preventing Malpractice on Long Term Care: Strategies for Risk Management*. New York: Springer Publishing Company.

Kapp, M.B. (1988). *Legal Aspects of Health Care for the Elderly: An Annotated Bibliography*. Westport, Conn: Greenwood Press.

Kapp, M.B., & Bigot, A. (1985). *Geriatrics and the Law: Patient Rights and Professional Responsibilities*. New York: Springer Publishing Company.

Kelly, G. (1951). The duty to preserve life. *Theological Studies, 12*(4):550–556.

Lynn, J. (1984). Food and water can be withheld from dying patients: The very different cases of Claire Conroy and Karen Quinlan. *Death Education, 8*(4):271–275.

Matter of Dinnerstein, 380 NE2d 134 (Mass App 1978).

Meisel, A. (1989). *The Right to Die*. New York: John Wiley & Sons.

Miles, S.H., & Gomez, C.F. (1989). *Protocols for Elective Use of Life-Sustaining Treatments*. New York: Springer Publishing Company.

Miller, R. (Speaker), & Bradley, L.M. (Producer). (1988). *Conflicts in Caring: Medical, Ethical, and Legal Perspectives in Bioethical Decision-Making* [Videotape]. Kansas City, Mo: Sheed and Ward.

Nolan, K. (1987). In death's shadow: The meanings of withholding resuscitation. *Hastings Center Report 17*(5):9–14.

Office of Technology Assessment. (July, 1987). *Life-Sustaining Technologies and the Elderly* (OTA-BA-306). Office of Technology Assessment. Washington, DC: US Government Printing Office.

O'Neil, E.A. (1987). Legal issues. In D. Lerman (Ed.) *Home Care: Positioning the Hospital for the Future*. Chicago: American Hospital Publishing, Inc.

O'Rourke, K.D., & Brodeur, D. (1989). *Medical Ethics: Common Ground for Understanding*. St. Louis: The Catholic Health Association.

Paris, J.J. (1986). When burdens of feeding outweigh benefits. *Hastings Center Report, 16*(1):30–32.

Parry, J. (1988). Selected recommendations from the national guardianship symposium at Wingspread. *Mental and Physical Disability Law Reporter, 12*(5): 398–406.

President's Commission for the Study of Ethical Problems in Medicine and Biomedical and Behavioral Sciences (1983). *Deciding to Forego Life-Sustaining Treatment: Ethical, Medical, and Legal Issues in Treatment Decisions*. Washington, DC: US Government Printing Office.

Appendix 4. Natural Death Acts

Ala Code §§22-8A-1 to 22-8A-10 (1984)
Alaska Stat §§18.12.010-.100 (1986)
Ariz Rev Stat Ann §§36-3201 to 36-3210 (1986)
Ark Stat Ann §§20-17-201 to 20-17-218 (Supp 1987)
Cal Health & Safety Code §§7185-7195 (West Supp 1988)
Colo Rev Stat §§15-18-101 to 15-18-113 (1987)
Conn Gen Stat Ann §§19a-570 to 19a-575 (West Supp 1988)
Del Code Ann §§Tit 16, 2501-2509 (1983)
DC Code Ann §§6-2421 to 6-2430 (Supp 1987)
Fla Stat Ann §§765.01-1.5 (West 1986)
Ga Code Ann §§31-31-1 to 31-32-12 (1985 & Supp 1988)
Hawaii Rev Stat §§327D-1 to 327D-27 (Supp 1987)
Idaho Code §§39-4502 to 39-4509 (Supp 1988)
Ill Ann Stat §§Ch 110 1/2 701-710 (Smith-Hurd Supp 1988)
Ind Code Ann §§16-8-11-1 to 16-8-22 (Burns Supp 1988)
Iowa Code Ann §§144A.1-.11 (West Supp 1988)
Kan Stat Ann §§65-28,101 to 65-28,109 (1985)
La Rev Stat Ann §§40:1299.58.1-.10 (West Supp 1988)
Me Rev Stat Ann Tit 22, §§2921-2931 (Supp 1987)
Md Health-Gen Code Ann §§5-601 to 5-614 (Supp 1987)
Minn §§5.28 (signed by Governor 3/3/89)
Miss Code Ann §§41-41-101 to 41-41-121 (Supp 1987)
Mo Ann Stat §§459.010-.055 (Vernon Supp 1988)
Mont Code Ann §§50-9-101 to 50-9-206 (1987)
Nev Rev Stat Ann §§449.540-.690 (Michie 1986)
NH Rev Stat Ann §§137-H:1 to 137-H:10 (Supp 1987)

NM Stat Ann §§24-7-1 to 24-7-11 (1986)
NC Gen Stat §§90-320 to 90-323 (1985)
ND HB §§1481 (1989)
Okla Stat Ann Tit 63, §§3101-3111 (West Supp 1988)
Or Rev Stat §§97.050-.090 (1985)
SC Code Ann §§44-77-10 to 44-77-160 (Law Co-op Supp 1987)
Tenn Code Ann §§32-11-101 to 32-11-110 (Supp 1988)
Tex Rev Civ Stat Ann Art 4590h §§1-11 (Vernon Supp 1988)
Utah Code Ann §§75-2-1101 to 75-2-1118 (Supp 1988)
Vt Stat Ann §§Tit 18, 5251-5262 (1987)
Va Code §§54-325.8:1-:13 (Supp 1987)
Wash Rev Code Ann §§70.122.010-105 (Supp 1987)
WVa Code §§16-30-1 to 16-30-10 (1985)
Wisc Stat Ann §§154.01-15 (West Supp 1987)
Wyo Stat §§33-26-144 to 33-26-152 (Supp 1987)

Chapter 5

Economics and Ethics

Amy Marie Haddad
Steven S. Martin

Case 5–1. The Wandering Client
Case 5–2. Hospital Versus Home Care Costs
Case 5–3. A Dying Client's Last Wish
Case 5–4. The Demanding Couple

The home care industry has grown and changed dramatically since the passage of Medicare (Title XVIII of the Social Security Act) in 1965. Not only has it grown regarding the number and variety of Medicare-certified providers, but it has grown in the number of clients served, services provided, and hours of care provided (Spohn, Bergthold, & Estes, 1988). With this growth, concerns have also increased regarding reimbursement for direct and indirect service delivery, access to home care services, and allocation of federal and private funds for home care as an alternative to acute or extended institutional care.

All of these concerns have an economic and ethical dimension. On the economic side, the concerns deal with efficiency and financial survival; on the ethical side, the concerns center around the principles of justice (what is fair) and beneficence (the duty to do good). There are far too many economic issues in home care to deal with all of them in this chapter. Therefore, this chapter focuses on selected economic issues that are most urgent in home care including allocation of health care dollars on a societal basis, regulatory restrictions, noncovered services, the burden of paper work, and the care of clinically needy but medically indigent clients. The ethical concerns and economic issues are discussed simultaneously, as neither can be entirely separated from the other.

ETHICAL ISSUES IN HOME CARE ECONOMICS

Home care providers have become expert at living with uncertainty. Medicare-certified providers have had to deal with a plethora of amendments and interpretations of the home care regulations since their inception. Home care providers on the private side have had to deal with numerous third-party payers and as many types of plans and contracts. In addition to uncertainty, home care providers have dealt with limits on reimbursement and the type and extent of services they can offer to clients.

> We must remember, however, that limits have always existed. At one time or another, healthcare has been short of physicians, nurses, hospitals, hospital beds, bandages, insurance, penicillin, and other resources. (Friedman, 1989, p. 32)

There have always been limits in home care but those that have developed in the last decade were not anticipated by providers or policy makers. A discussion of limits necessarily leads to the broader issue of allocation of health care resources. "To allocate is to distribute resources among alternative uses" (Veatch, 1989, p. 294). It is helpful to explore the question of allocation on two levels: societal and individual.

Societal Allocation Issues

As a society, we collectively decide how we will spend our resources in health care and other areas such as education or defense. This type of allocation decision is on a larger scale than a decision by a home care nurse to spend more time with Mrs. Donahoe on a home visit even though it means spending less time with Mrs. Strunk. Therefore, the distinction between societal and individual allocation decisions seems to rest on the level at which the decision is being made and the amount of resources being considered. Some consider this distinction misleading, as it gives the impression that there is some sort of organized system for making allocation decisions in health care.

> Whether or not any existing society is in fact this highly structured in its mechanism for allocation may be a matter of controversy, but it is fair to say that the United States, perhaps more so than many industrialized countries, currently lacks anything that could realistically be called an allocation system with regard to health-care resources. (Veatch, 1989, p. 295)

In the United States, it is evident that the majority of our health care resources go to acute care, largely in the form of intensive, crisis-oriented medicine. On the positive side, this focus in health care priorities assists those individuals who will directly benefit from crisis intervention. On the down side, it is the most expensive form of care and reaches fewer clients, with generally less favorable prognoses.

The emphasis on and support of high technology, crisis-intervention medicine limits what can be accomplished in preventive and long-term care. In addition, chronically ill clients often do not need or use the resources available in the acute care hospital. "Even in situations of abundant resources, cost of care may be unnecessarily increased if resources continue to be made available to patients who could be cared for elsewhere equally well or at lower cost" (Bergner et al, 1988, p. 566). Yet, there has been only a slight effort to shift resources to alternative delivery models of health care.

Questions of allocation are never as simple as an "either/or" proposition. What if we continue to spend as we have on crisis-intervention health care? What if we shifted our focus to less technical, long-term care services? Persons 85 years old and older are the fastest growing segment of our population (Watts & McCally, 1984). Should we therefore allocate the lion's share of our resources to the long-term care services this population will certainly need? What exactly are "long-term care services?" What the health professions and society face, then, are decisions that must weigh the maximum cost efficiency of allocations against the needs of individuals, as well as decisions that must strike some kind of reasonable and justifiable balance between crisis-oriented health care and long-term care services (personal care and social supportive services) both in and out of the home (Barry, 1982).

In the last decade, the expansion of home care services has been enhanced by Congressional and administrative policy. Federal attempts to constrain the spending of acute care hospitals and efforts to reduce dependence on institutional long-term care have clearly led to the promotion of home care as an effective, less costly alternative. Though this is true, it has not resulted in any significant decrease in hospital care and nursing home care, which together still account for over half of health care expenditures.

Home health care has increased, but it still comprises only 3 percent of overall Medicare costs. Even before the introduction of prospective payment for Medicare hospital patients, the number of home care clients was increasing at a rate of over 10 percent annually (Benjamin, 1986). From 1974 to 1980 Medicare expenditures for home care increased at an annual rate of 34 percent. However, Medicare coverage and reimbursement policies for home care have resulted in less sizable increases during the 1980s. Notably, Medicare spending for home health care increased only 4.3 percent in 1986 and 6.4 percent in 1987 (Curtiss, 1988).

However, it is important to note the relative value of this amazing growth in the home care industry.

> In contrast to the rapid increase in utilization, increases in reimbursement per visit and the reimbursement per person has been more modest. While reimbursement per visit did grow at over 9 percent per

> year between 1974 and 1982, after accounting for the rate of inflation in the economy at large, the actual rate of increase was only 0.5 percent per year. (Bishop & Stassen, 1986, p. 19)

Therefore, it is obvious that the unprecedented growth in home care is not due to profits from service delivery. One must also consider the profits in the product area of home care, which account for the bulk of economic growth. Home infusion therapy ventures have been among the most profitable in health care (Lutz, 1989). The growth of medical home care equipment is expected to increase dramatically through the next decade. It is far easier to make a profit from a product than it is from a human service. All of the various funding sources for home care make a clear distinction between product and service reimbursement.

Sources of Funding. While public funding for home care remains minimal compared to expenditures for acute care and institutional long-term care, public funding has played a key role in shaping home care services. There are several funding sources that, because of their separate target populations, eligibility requirements, and separate administration, have tended to increase the fragmentation of home care services (US Congress, 1986).

The primary federal funding source for the home care industry as a whole is Medicare. Medicare provides more than 70 percent of Medicare-certified home health care agency revenues (Balinsky & Starkman, 1987). Under the Medicare home health benefit, reimbursement is provided for the care of homebound Medicare-eligible beneficiaries in need of part-time or intermittent skilled nursing, physical therapy, or speech therapy. Except for a 20 percent co-pay for durable medical equipment, the Medicare recipient pays no deductible and no co-pay for Part A home health services. The Health Care Financing Administration (HCFA) administers the Medicare program at the federal level.

Medicaid, Title XIX of the Social Security act, is a state administered program but is jointly funded by both state and federal governments. It is designed to meet the medical and rehabilitative needs of low-income individuals (individuals who meet the poverty guidelines in each state) who are blind, disabled, or over 65 years of age. Since it is a state-run program, there is considerable discretion over coverage and eligibility requirements. However, states have followed Medicare's lead in setting service levels, eligibility and provider criteria, and reimbursement methods (Spohn, Bergthold, & Estes, 1988).

Medicaid expenditures for home care services account for less than 2 percent of the Medicaid budget nationally. Medicaid home health services are not widely utilized and are primarily limited to personal care services received in less than half of the states.

While Medicare is the largest payer of home care services through Part A funding of professional and personal caregivers and Part B funding of supplies, equipment, and total parenteral nutrition solutions, other payers have followed Medicare's lead in payment approaches to home care. Private insurance funds have, to varying degrees, copied the Medicare model of paying for intermittent skilled nursing services and therapies. Most private payers are more restrictive. Also, insurance plans generally cover younger populations (under 65) who have less demand for home care services than the more fragile, over-65 Medicare population. Very few private insurance plans pay for personal care services, such as home health aide services. Most private insurers pay for home medical equipment, supplies, and intravenous solutions in a manner similar to Medicare.

Finally, clients and their families can pay directly for home care services. The amount of direct client payments for home care is hard to estimate but is thought to be substantial.

It is important to note that in health care financing, regardless of whether the source is federal or private, it has always been easier to recover reimbursement for medical products and equipment than for personal or professional services. This has been particularly problematic for the home care industry, as it is fundamentally a service industry.

Ethical Impact of Regulatory Restrictions. At the state or regional level, Medicare is administered by 10 geographically dispersed fiscal intermediaries (FIs). FIs are HCFA contractors that monitor provider performance. FIs are responsible for: (1) making payments to certified home health agencies; (2) serving as communication linkages between HCFA and the agencies; and (3) serving as gatekeepers and safeguards against inappropriate use of program services (Benjamin, 1986).

There is a great degree of variability in performance review among the FIs. This variability has given rise to numerous complaints by home care providers and clients. The essence of these complaints can be distilled to the following three issues:

- The inconsistent administration and interpretation of the home health benefit among intermediaries.
- The increased denial rates of intermediaries.
- The slowdown in payments made by intermediaries. (Christiansen, 1987)

For example, the statutory language in Title XVIII does not clearly define "intermittent care" or "homebound." Therefore, the FIs can interpret this statutory intent with great latitude. The following case illustrates the impact of a strict interpretation of the "homebound" requirement.

Case 5–1. The Wandering Client

Dr. Griffin is a retired internist. He practiced medicine for over 45 years before he was forced to retire because of a multitude of health problems. Dr. Griffin has diabetes, congestive heart failure, chronic pulmonary disease, and Alzheimer's disease. He falls frequently and needs the assistance of his wife, a visiting nurse, and a respiratory therapist. Further, he has daily periods of extreme confusion during which he becomes quite agitated, to the point of striking out at his wife.

His care was denied by the FI as not covered because he failed to meet the requirements of being confined to his home. This decision was based on the 485 and 486 forms that were submitted. In the context of explaining significant clinical findings, the nurse noted the following incident. Mrs. Griffin called the home care agency in a panic state. She reported that Dr. Griffin had become extremely agitated and confused and had pushed her down. She had lost consciousness for a brief period of time and when she came to, Dr. Griffin was not in the house. Mrs. Griffin had developed an elaborate set of locks on all of the doors and yet Dr. Griffin was able to escape. The nurse encouraged Mrs. Griffin to call the police.

Mrs. Griffin did so. Six hours later, the police found Dr. Griffin huddled in a doorway of a downtown business office. Evidently, he had gotten on a bus and ridden until the driver made him get off. He had wandered around downtown until it got dark. Dr. Griffin was very confused, exhausted, and cold. Other parts of the nurse's notes indicated that Dr. Griffin could not be left alone; that clearly there was a need to keep him in the home; and that he and his wife lived alone.

This discretionary power to interpret the intent of the Medicare regulations has clear ethical implications. First, in order to be fairly administered, the regulations must be uniformly interpreted. The Social Security Act [Section 1861v(1)] states that Medicare beneficiaries are entitled to reimbursement for all medically reasonable and necessary care. Any limitations of this entitlement must be based on a rational, nonarbitrary cost methodology or a demonstrated, published clinical determination regarding the medical necessity and reasonableness of particular treatments (Randall, 1987). It is clear that the regulations are not uniformly administered and, therefore, beneficiaries are not receiving fair treatment.

Justice refers to giving everyone his or her due. "One acts justly toward a person when that person has been given what is due or owed, and thus what he or she deserves and can legitimately claim" (Beauchamp & Childress, 1983, p. 184). Therefore, if a Medicare recipient deserves home care services as described in the regulations and receives those services, justice has been done. In the case of Dr. Griffin, it would seem obvious that he met the "homebound" requirement. The regulations state, ". . . a patient with a psychiatric problem (meets the homebound requirement) if his illness is manifested in part by a refusal to leave his home environment or is of such nature that it would not be considered safe for him to leave his home unattended, even if he has no physical limitations" (Health Care Financing Administration, 1989, Section 204.1A).

Second, narrow interpretations of the regulations can and do result in real harm to the individuals who need the services the most. The harm that results takes a variety of forms: denial of benefits, a reluctance of home care providers to take cases that are questionable or likely to be denied, the harms that can result from lack of services or discontinuance of needed services, and spending more time on documentation than client care. It is clear in Dr. Griffin's case that he and his wife would not be able to continue to live safely for very long in their home without the support of home care services.

In addition to the inconsistent interpretation of home health benefits, Dr. Griffin's case indicates the problem of increased rates of denial by intermediaries. Approximately 6 percent of home health care claims are being denied by Medicare, and it is estimated that this will increase to 8 percent before it will decrease (Droste, 1987). The performance of FIs is reviewed by HCFA. One of the performance critera that FIs are evaluated by is referred to as the "5-to-1" policy.

> Under this policy, fiscal intermediaries are required to find $5 in "erroneous" coverage allowances for every $1 spent in reviewing home health agency decisions. Apparently no provision is made for finding erroneous coverage denials by a home health agency. (Komlos-Hrobsky & Vail, 1987, p. 32)

The pressures created by a system such as this probably do more harm to clients than restriction of eligibility standards. The FIs are encouraged to find individuals who were "erroneously" granted benefits. On the surface, a policy that encourages the elimination of waste is ethically correct, as it is then possible to make the best use of scarce resources. However, the "5-to-1" policy is not ethically sound because it may encourage denials at a set rate even if no legitimate reasons for a denial exist so that FIs can meet HCFAs' performance standards and retain their contracts.

Recent legal action initiated by the home care industry has brought about significant changes in the clarification of eligibility requirements. The landmark ruling in the *Duggan v Bowen* (1988) suit established a policy defining "part-time or intermittent" care. The court approved the proposed policy, which involves a calculation of a client's entitlement to coverage based on hours of service in a week. The decision permits daily home care services. Clients are now eligible for payment of necessary nursing and home health aide services up to thirty-five hours a week regardless of the number of days a week that care is provided. Extension of coverage beyond thirty-five hours will also be available in exceptional circumstances.

In human terms, this single decision will have a ripple effect throughout the lives of numerous Medicare beneficiaries. The clinical reality of shorter lengths of stay in the hospital has increased the need for extended home care services immediately following hospital discharge. This is particularly true in the case of the frail elderly who are the most vulnerable and therefore the most at risk.

Selling a Product or a Service. Though significant progress has been made in the past decade in the struggle to clarify the meaning, intent, and fair administration of the Medicare home health program, home care providers have spent far less time on internal issues that are extremely important to the growth of the industry. While the battles with HCFA and the FIs have been raging, the home care industry has lacked cohesion and has lagged behind in the development of the business side of care. There is a clear need for research that will document whom home care providers are treating, at what frequency of service, and at what cost (Randall, 1987). This type of data is essential to the further growth of the industry.

It is difficult to define home care because it encompasses so many types of services and products, which can run the gamut from short- to long-term; from medical to supportive social services (nursing, social work, rehabilitation, home health aide/homemaker, and other personal care services) that supplement, complement, or substitute for institutional care (Shamansky, 1988).

Regarding the outcome of home care service delivery, the findings from several studies are inconsistent as to the cost-savings of home care, though reduced cost is often promoted as one of the primary benefits of home care. The costs of home care for such diverse diagnoses as the need for ventilatory support in children and adults and home infusion therapies (antimicrobial therapy, parenteral nutrition, analgesic and rehydration therapy) have been compared to equivalent costs of hospitalization. In most cases, home care resulted in significant costs savings (Aday, Wegener, Anderson, & Aitken, 1989; Culbertson, Rhodes, Hill, & Rhodes, 1988; Gentry, 1988; Motwani & Herring, 1988).

Home care does not always yield costs savings. Bergner et al (1988) found that in the case of clients with chronic lung disease who were not at immediate risk of institutionalization, home care services provided in a more liberal fashion did not appear to produce cost savings nor did they seem to enhance everyday functioning or mental state.

In addition, nonpecuniary costs must also be weighed in the analysis. In the case of ventilator-dependent children, the greater the extent of professional nursing in the home, the lower the costs savings (Aday et al, 1989). However, even though the costs were less in families who had less professionl nursing support, the families felt unprepared for the burdens of care delivery. These "costs" included feelings of abandonment and isolation (Aday et al, 1989).

Generally speaking, home care incurs lower costs than would be incurred during an equivalent stay in the hospital. This is most often true on the service side of home care. It is not always true on the product side, as is evidenced in the following case.

Case 5–2. Hospital versus Home Care Costs

Nancy Abbott lived in a midsize midwest city and was 3 months pregnant with her second child. For the last week she had not been able to stop vomiting long enough to keep any food down. When she became too weak to lift her head off the pillow, her husband took her to the emergency room where she was met by her obstetrician. Dr. Bettis wrote the following diagnosis on the clinical record, "Hyperemesis gravidarum." Dr. Bettis ordered the following: "Lactated Ringer's solution, 1000 cc to run at 2 mL/min over eight hours." Dr. Bettis was about to write the order to admit Nancy to the hospital when Nancy asked if she could receive the intravenous fluids at home. Dr. Bettis felt home care would be appropriate in this case so she changed the order to read: "Lactated Ringer's solution, 2 liters to run at 3 mL/min followed by 1 liter at HS (bedtime) at 2 mL/min per heparin lock for the next three nights."

A home infusion therapy company called Our Town Home Care was called in by Dr. Bettis. A heparin lock was inserted in the emergency room and Nancy returned home and received the intravenous solutions without any complications. Her symptoms subsided and she did not require any further intravenous therapy.

The Our Town Home Care Company, which supplied the solutions and equipment for Nancy's care, submitted the following claim to Nancy's private insurer. The charges for the 5 liters of Ringer's lactate, intravenous tubing, and filters were $900.00, rental for the intravenous pole $50.00, and rental for an infusion pump $450.00. Total charges for the solutions, tubing, and equipment rental was $1400.00. The Our Town Home Care Company had an agreement with the local visiting nurse association to deliver skilled nursing care. The visiting nurse association submitted a claim to the insurance company for three skilled visits at $65.00 per visit, or a total of $195.00. The total charges submitted to the company for Nancy's home care were $1595.00.

The insurance company's claims auditor who processed this claim contacted a local wholesale medical supplier to determine actual wholesale costs. She discovered that lactated Ringer's solution costs approximately $5.00 per liter and the average retail markup was $33.00 per liter. She also discovered that the purchase cost of a new infusion pump and pole was approximately $2000.00. Nancy's insurance company was a traditional insurance plan that had no restrictions on where Nancy sought care. They had no contractual agreement limiting Our Town Home Care on what they could charge, so the insurer was required to pay the charges according to the insurance contract. Nancy's insurance covered 100 percent of inpatient care after a deductible of $100.00 and covered 80 percent of all outpatient care and equipment. The out-of-pocket cost to Nancy for care given by Our Town Home Care and the Visiting Nurse Association was 20 percent of the total charge, or $319.00.

The cost of Nancy's care for three days in a local hospital would have been $1200.00 or 24 percent less than the home care charge and would have cost Nancy $100.00 instead of $319.00. The cost of Nancy's care in a skilled nursing facility would have been $395.00, or 75 percent less than the cost of home care. Also, in this case, Nancy's family was required to take on a greater caregiver role. Nancy's husband had never seen an infusion pump before and was instructed by the visiting nurse regarding its operation and safe management. Because of his concern for his wife and fear of something going wrong with the equipment, he did not sleep for the three nights Nancy received infusion therapy.

This was only one case, but it was a case that the insurance company would not forget. Unlike hospital and physician claims, home health claims are generally open to 100 percent review for medical necessity. Therefore, home health claims are subject to greater scrutiny. A case such as this proved to the insurance company that home care was not a predictable, cost-effective alternative to institutional care.

> Most private insurance programs now have better mechanisms for responding to requests for determinations of coverage of home health services, but home care is still viewed primarily as a substitute for inpatient care rather than as a medical benefit that is explicitly

covered under group and individual insurance policies. (Curtiss, 1988, p. 1682)

When the insurance company evaluates its benefit schedule they will remember the charges for this case. It is unlikely that the insurer would expand home care benefits to broader coverage because they could rightfully anticipate the same sort of unpredictable charges from other suppliers.

With the exception of the Medicare hospice program, there is no national model for delivery of home care services that requires one provider to coordinate and ensure the reasonable use of resources. In Nancy Abbott's case, who was responsible for ensuring the appropriate use of resources? Should Nancy have inquired as to the cost of home care services while she was in the emergency room? Was the physician responsible for advising Nancy on the financial burdens of her choices? Was the insurance company responsible for advising Nancy in advance of her care? Should the insurance company have had a contractual agreement with Our Town Home Care or another similar company to ensure the cost while limiting Nancy's choice of provider? What is fair remuneration for health care products as opposed to health care services?

This case illustrates the inequities between service and product suppliers in home care. The case may appear extreme or the norm depending on the competitive environment in a given community. There is a great disparity between service and product operating margins, which can account for some of the inequities. It is hard to make a profit when a home care provider is being reimbursed for services only.

This is the sort of dilemma that the Medicare program and some private insurers attempted to resolve when they established maximum fee schedules. In order to control for wide variations in charges, maximum fee schedules for supplies and durable medical equipment are set across the board, which has resulted in reduced payments. The home care product industry, on the other hand, has argued that cases like the Nancy Abbott case are exceptions and limiting payments may limit both the quality of service and access and availability by reducing competitors in some marketplaces. Durable medical equipment suppliers have experienced what they perceive to be relentless cutbacks in Medicare reimbursement rates and often have faced cash-flow difficulties as a result of slow claims payments (ninety days or longer in many areas of the country)(Bryant, 1987). Long receivable delays and lowest-charge-level methods could result in cost shifting to private payers. This has been a common practice in the acute care setting but in the long run results in increased costs to all payers.

Individual Allocation Issues

While the home care industry collectively works to increase home care's market share, nurses and therapists must contend with the more personal allocation issues that they encounter daily. Home health agency administrators and personnel must deal with some very basic questions of justice such as: Who gets what when not all have enough? How do we decide fairly?

Non-covered Services. As the face of home care has changed, so has the type of services provided to clients and families. Clients are generally more complex and require more types of services in order to stay in their homes. This results in a greater need for coordination of the members of the home care team. Coordination, or the concept of case management, has been used in a variety of ways by different health care disciplines. Case management includes assessment, planning, implementation, and evaluation on a variety of interpersonal and interprofessional levels. The goals of case management are quality care, reduced fragmentation of services, the enhancement of the client's quality of life, and the containment of costs (American Nurses' Association, 1988).

However, just like home care in general, case management does not always result in cost savings. Case management may in fact increase the cost of care because clients are exposed to a wider array of services and therefore use them more. Case management must be encouraged on the basis of not only cost containment but the benefits accrued by clients and their families.

Case management involves a number of activities over the course of a day and a case. The following case illustrates the myriad activities that are necessary to safely take a complex client home.

Case 5–3. A Dying Client's Last Wish

Allison Addams was dying of metastatic cancer of the liver. She was no longer a viable candidate for any type of treatment. Though Allison was only 56 years old, she was a widow. After her husband's death, she moved into an efficiency apartment to "get away from the memories." Allison's husband had died of cancer of the lung. Allison told her physician, "I saw how Harold died surrounded by tubes and machines. I don't want that. I don't want to die in the hospital, but I don't want to die alone in my apartment either." Allison's only relative was her older sister, Marge, also a widow, who lived in Fairbury, a small rural community approximately 45 miles from the hospital. After visiting with Allison one day, Marge told the physician, "I would be willing to take Allison home with me if it could be arranged."

Since by this time death appeared imminent, there was a flurry of activity to find a home care provider who was willing to take the case. Allison's care consisted of pain management with morphine via an ambulatory pump, basic physical care, and support. Super Care Home Care agreed to assess Allison's case. Eileen O'Reilly, the nursing supervisor for Super Care, visited Allison in the hospital. Eileen spoke with Allison regarding her expectations of home care. Allison was particularly lucid during the assessment visit and was able to tell Eileen that she knew she would die soon, that she did not want any aggressive measures to be taken to change that fact, and that she really wanted to get out of the hospital as soon as possible.

Eileen read Allison's chart, consulted with the primary nurse and other staff nurses who had made entries on Allison's hospital care plan, and called the physician to discuss his perspective on the case. Eileen then called Marge to arrange a home visit in order to assess the suitability of the home environment.

After the home visit, Eileen felt she had enough data to determine that Super Care could take Allison home safely. Eileen met with Allison and Marge and a service agreement was secured contingent on insurance coverage. Allison understood that if she stayed in the hospital, her costs would be completely covered. Neither Allison nor Marge had the financial resources to pay directly for home care services, particularly if Allison lived longer than anticipated.

Eileen then called Allison's private insurer to see if home care services would be covered. She found that Allison's insurer had the ability to waive contractual benefits and authorize home care services as an alternative to hospitalization. However, the insurer required a proposal for the waiver that included verification of the medical necessity of the care, the method of care delivery, the coordinated role of the providers, goals for treatment outcomes, and the cost savings.

Super Care had dealt with this insurer before and therefore had developed proposal materials that could be quickly assembled for presentation to the insurer. Eileen prepared the proposal and submitted it to the insurer in person in order to expedite the review process. Two days later, Allison's insurer called Super Care to let them know the proposal had been approved. The insurer would cover twelve hours of skilled nursing service a day for thirty days.

While the insurer was reviewing the proposal, Eileen had been organizing the care plan for the case and the necessary staff. Since the case was 45 miles away from Super Care's office, Eileen attempted to hire nurses in Fairbury. Eileen ran an advertisement in the local newspaper and called the nursing home and hospital in Fairbury for potential leads. Eileen was able to come up with four nurses who were willing to work on the case. However, none of the nurses had ever worked in home care or even seen an ambulatory infusion pump.

Eileen contacted Allison's physician for a treatment plan and then finalized the care plan. She also arranged for an in-service orientation by the infusion therapy company that was assigned to the case and would supply the infusion pump and medications. The four nurses from Fairbury were paid by Super Care Home Care for four hours of orientation to the infusion pump, medications, and the general plan of care.

All of this preparation took five days to coordinate. This was not the only case that Eileen was working on either. The afternoon of the fourth day after the initial assessment visit, Allison was able to be discharged to her sister's home in Fairbury. Allison died comfortably in her sister's home three days later.

While it is true that indirect nursing clinical case management activities are, to some degree, reimbursed as part of the indirect administrative overhead costs, the fact remains that under the present system of payment for services, which is usually on a per visit basis, the home care provider stands to lose financially on cases such as Allison's. Super Care Home Care invested approximately $920.00 in staff salaries, mileage, and orientation wages preparing for Allison's case. They provided thirty-six hours of home care at $25.00 per hour charge. This provided Super Care Home Care with a 30 percent operating margin or a total operating profit of $270.00. This still leaves Super Care Home Care with a $650 dollar loss on this case. Allison would have had to survive for ten days in order for Super Care Home Care to recover its initial investment. There are no guarantees in a case like Allison's. Is this the best way to conduct a home care business? Other businesses plan for risks and deal with losses like this by using volume to project gains and losses over time. If a home care provider in a community has a low volume of this type of case, it would not be financially prudent for it to take a case such as Allison's.

Home care providers and third-party payers should examine the methods of planning for home care and attempt to find effective business strategies to cover front end costs of home care planning and case management. If this were done, home care providers would be able to establish hourly costs at a reasonable and predictable rate for services provided.

There are other issues at work in this case besides the financial stability of the home care provider. Distributive justice refers to the justified distribution of burdens and benefits in society. "Justice is comparative when what one person deserves can be determined only by balancing the competing claims of other persons against his or her claims" (Beauchamp & Childress, 1983, p. 185). Problems such as these only arise under conditions of scarcity and competition. If there were adequate reimbursement for home care services and all home care providers in a community that agreed to share equally the burden of the care of the medically indigent, compliance with the principles of distributive justice would be simple.

Super Care Home Care had to weigh the following alternatives in Allison's case: there was a significant chance that Allison would not live long enough for them to recover their investment; despite this chance, it would have been an injustice not to allow Allison to die at home; and Super Care wanted to establish themselves in the marketplace as a home care provider with integrity, one willing to take the good with the bad.

Such a weighing of alternatives, especially of risks and benefits, is typical of problems of distributive justice. A more basic question in this case deals with the need for home care. Did Allison need home care? The principle of need declares that distribution is fair when it is based on need. A person is in need of something if without it the person will be harmed (or at least detrimentally affected)(Beauchamp & Childress, 1983). In Allison's case, no discernible physical harm would have occurred if she had not been able to return home. However, there is the issue of emotional and psychological harm that is particularly compelling in the case of a dying client. Super Care responded to Allison's need and was willing to accept the risk of a moderate financial loss. Super Care responded in a humane fashion to the request of a terminally ill, vulnerable person. There is a sort of moral intuition at work here that goes beyond what is fair.

> The rudimentary character of this moral knowledge that those in need must be aided is such that it is as likely a concern of charity as it is a consideration of justice. With this starting point, charity plays two roles. It is coextensive with justice, enlivening it and preventing retreat into empty abstractions. And it is larger than justice, setting goals beyond those that rights alone require. (Dougherty, 1989, p. 131)

Another activity that is not directly covered by reimbursement is the paper work required to get reimbursement. The incredible amount of paper work in home care causes a classic dilemma. On the one hand, home care providers, particularly nurses and direct caregivers, value hands-on care and the time they spend with clients and families. On the other hand, if the care is not accurately documented, the provider will not be reimbursed. Accurate documentation takes time. Therefore, more time must be spent on documentation, which leaves less time for client care.

It is not likely that the amount and depth of documentation will decrease in the near future. Numerous tactics have been suggested to deal with this dilemma, such as decreasing non-nursing functions, documenting care on site, decreasing unnecessary repetition in records, and time studies to determine reasonable productivity (Morrissey-Ross, 1988). On a wider basis, home care providers must work to decrease record keeping requirements that are threatening the fundamental purpose of home care—client care.

Discontinuing Care to Nonpaying, Needy Clients. In Allison's case, the home care provider knew that it was going to be reimbursed for the services it delivered, though there was no guarantee that the amount would cover the initial investment. Nurses and home care administrators are faced with many other cases in which reimbursement is not possible at all or has been discontinued. This assumes that the home care provider exhausted all forms of community and federal sources of reimbursement. Does the nurse or the home care provider have an obligation to continue home care when there is no reimbursement?

In American society there is no guaranteed legal right to health care for all citizens. Specific groups may have an entitlement to specific health care services or insurance, but on the whole the provider is under no obligation to provide care without reimbursement. The only case in which an obligation does exist is in the case of emergency care. If a client is in a life-threatening situtation, the nurse or other home care professional has a clear moral and legal obligation to secure adequate institutional care.

The more common and more problematic cases are those in which the home care provider has established a caring relationship with the client and then reaches a point where funding is exhausted or denied. The client is in no immediate danger but still is in need of home care services.

> The problem lies in the differing interpretations of minimum standards of care by funding sources and by professional nurses. Individual and societal consequences of providing care while imperiling the agency are difficult to measure. Declaring one consequence superior to another in terms of respect for human dignity is therefore impossible. (Reckling, 1989, p. 79)

As has been discussed elsewhere (see Chapter 9), the home care provider may discontinue care without abandoning the client. Though the home care provider is not ethically obligated to continue care to medically indigent clients, there is a broader obligation to public policy planners and society. There is a professional responsibility to let individuals who have an impact on health policy decisions know that care is being denied to needy people because of lack of funding. This places an additional burden on home care providers to distinguish between needed and desired services and to identify the impact of denial of needed services in concrete, outcome-based terms.

Discontinuing Care to Paying Clients. It would be inappropriate to suggest that home care providers are primarily concerned with reimbursement to the exclusion of providing quality care. Quite the contrary is true. In many cases, when it is obvious that services do not have the potential for reimbursement, nurses and other providers attempt to maintain the quality of care by concentrating services into a shorter period of time (Harris, 1989).

There are cases in which reimbursement is not the issue, where in fact, reimbursement is guaranteed for an extended period of time at an acceptable market rate. Yet, there still can be conflicts between the client's expectations and the provider's ability to provide the service. This is patently obvious in the following case.

Case 5–4. The Demanding Couple

Cecil "King" Benson and his wife, May, are well known by all the home care providers in the community. King is 82 years old, blind, and has a permanent colostomy. King also has rheumatoid arthritis and needs assistance with all of his activities of daily living, which include shaving, bathing, irrigation, changing and cleansing of his colostomy, dressing, ambulation, and meal preparation. May, at 80, is in equally bad shape but is able to see and ambulate with only a moderate degree of assistance.

The Bensons are well known because they have been to almost every home care provider in the community for home health aide services. The Bensons are financially well-off and can afford to pay for any type of home care services they need. They have turned to the home care agencies in the past, since they have had little luck in retaining the aides they have hired privately.

It seems that nothing is ever quite right according to the Bensons' standards. Each home health provider has run through its roster of aides, but no aide has lasted more than a week. Either the aide is too slow or too fast, makes lumpy oatmeal or gets the eggs too brown, doesn't shave King correctly or uses the wrong linens to change the beds. King gets physically agitated and strikes out at the aides when he doesn't like the care he's receiving and May verbally berates them. It has not been uncommon for an aide to ask to be removed from the Benson case before getting "fired" by May.

A few of the home care providers have suggested that the Bensons move into an extended care facility together. The Bensons have turned down that suggestion, stating flatly that they are happy in their home if only they could find "good help."

A-1 Home Care has recently agreed to take the Bensons on as clients. In the last 2 weeks, the Bensons have dismissed three of A-1's best home health aides. The home health aides have discussed the case among themselves and now A-1 is having difficulty getting an aide to agree to take the case. A-1 is, in a sense, the Bensons' last chance. There are no other home care providers to turn to in the community. When A-1 Home Care is finally unable to provide staffing for the Bensons because of staff refusals to work for the Bensons they will be forced to advise them of this limitation.

The home care provider has one last alternative to salvage the case. A-1 can provide additional clinical supervision of the home health aides to help defuse some of the difficulties. This extra supervision will cut into the approximately $3.00 per hour in total contribution to agency overhead. A-1 must weigh the burdens and benefits involved in continuing with the case or cutting its losses. Costs are not always measured only in dollars and cents. A-1 must also consider the time, energy, and aggravation involved in a case like this. Though the case is a guaranteed source of revenue, it may not be worth it in the long run to the home care provider and its staff.

After A-1 has made the decision to discontinue care, it should be completely clear with the Bensons about the differences in their respective expectations. If the quality of care provided by A-1 is not satisfactory to the Bensons, A-1 cannot fulfill its service agreement and therefore can discontinue services. A-1 could assist the Bensons in finding alternative services such as domestic help or a "live-in" by referring them to appropriate agencies and businesses within the community.

SUMMARY

The value of home care is real but difficult to measure. Home care providers are going to continue to be faced with the dual challenge of being proactive in shaping home health benefits and surviving in an economy in which new federal spending is limited because of the large federal deficit. Generally, the narrow operating margins in home care services raise serious questions about client benefit becoming a secondary consideration to the home care provider's survival. The home care provider may be tempted to place administrative or insurance company needs above those of the client. The rigidity of the current economic structure can be resolved through economic principles of cost consciousness meshed with quality client care. Economics and ethics are not contradictions in home care practice. Ethical analysis can help to identify and articulate the values within the home care industry that society wants to pursue. Economic structures can then facilitate society's ability to realize these values through ethically sound allocation principles and healthy economic structures (O'Rourke & Brodeur, 1989).

REFERENCES

Aday, L.A., Wegener, D.H., Anderson, R.M., & Aitken, M.J. (1989). Home care for ventilator-assisted children. *Health Affairs, 8*(2):137–147.

American Nurses' Association. (1988). *Nursing Case Management.* Report of the Task Force on Case Management in Nursing. Kansas City, Mo: American Nurses' Association.

Balinsky, W., & Starkman, J.L. (1987). The impact of DRGs on the health care industry. *Health Care Management Review, 12*(3):61–74.

Barry, V. (1982). *Moral Aspects of Health Care.* Belmont, Calif: Wadsworth Publishing Company.

Beauchamp, T.L., & Childress, J.F. (1983). *Principles of Biomedical Ethics* (2nd ed.) New York: Oxford University Press.

Benjamin, A.E. (1986). Trends and issues in the provision of home health care: Local governments in competitive environment. *Journal of Public Health Policy,* 7:480–494.

Bergner, M., Hudson, L.D., Conrad, D.A., Patmont, C.M., McDonald, G.J., Perrin, E.B., & Gilson, B.S. (1988). The cost and efficacy of home care for patients with chronic lung disease. *Medical Care, 26*:566–579.

Bishop, C., & Stassen, M. (1986). Prospective reimbursement for home health care: Context for an evolving policy. *PRIDE Institute Journal of Long Term Home Health Care, 5*(1):17–26.

Bryant, M. (1987, January 2). Home care profits shrink, costs rise under tighter Medicare rules. *Washington Report on Medicine and Health*, pp. 1–4.

Christiansen, K. (1987). The fiscal intermediary's role in administering the home health benefit. *PRIDE Institute Journal of Long Term Home Health Care, 6*(4):34–40.

Culbertson, V.L., Rhodes, R.S., Hill, E.P., & Rhodes, P.J. (1988). Impact of home infusion therapy on the Colorado Medicaid program budget. *American Journal of Hospital Pharmacy, 45*:1346–1349.

Curtiss, F. (1988). Recent developments in federal reimbursement for home health-care services and products. *American Journal of Hospital Pharmacy, 45*:1682–1690.

Dougherty, C. (1988). *American health care: Realities, rights, and reforms.* New York: Oxford University Press.

Droste, T. (1987, June 5). Alternate care: Medicare denials threaten the health of home care. *Hospitals*, p. 58.

Duggan v Bowen, 691 F Supp 1487 (D DC 1988).

Friedman, E. (1989). The weird new health care boat. *Health Progress, 70*(1):32–38.

Gentry, L.O. (1988). Home management of osteomyelitis. *Bulletin of the New York Academy of Medicine, 64*:565–569.

Harris, M.D. (1989). The impact of one federal regulation on productivity in a home health agency. *Home Healthcare Nurse, 7*(5):37–40.

Health Care Financing Administration (1989). *Medicare Home Health Agency Health Insurance Manual-11.* Washington, DC: US Government Printing Office.

Komlos-Hrobsky, P., & Vail, J. (1987). A legal services perspective on representing Medicare home health patients. *PRIDE Institute Journal of Long Term Home Health Care, 6*(4):26–33.

Lutz, S. (1989). Home care's growth hinges on winning over physicians. *Modern Healthcare, 19*(39):20–30.

Morrissey-Ross, M. (1988). Documentation: If you haven't written it, you haven't done it. *Nursing Clinics of North America, 23*:363–371.

Motwani, J.K., & Herring, G.M. (1988). Home care for ventilator-dependent persons: A cost-effective, humane public policy. *Health and Social Work, 13*(1):20–24.

O'Rourke, K.D., & Brodeur, D. (1989). *Medical ethics: Common ground for understanding.* St. Louis: The Catholic Health Association.

Randall, D.A. (1987). Home health services under Medicare: The need for organized responses to growth and change. *PRIDE Institute Journal for Long Term Home Health Care, 6*(4):3–18.

Reckling, J.B. (1989). Abandonment of patients by home health nursing agencies: An ethical analysis of the dilemma. *Advances in Nursing Science, 11*(3):70–81.

Shamansky, S.L. (1988). Providing home care services in a for-profit environment. *Nursing Clinics of North America, 23*:387–398.

Spohn, P.H, Bergthold, L., & Estes, C.L. (1988). From cottage to condos: The expansion of the home health care industry under Medicare. *Home Health Services Quarterly, 8*(4):25–55.

Veatch, R. (1989). *Medical Ethics.* Boston, Mass: Jones and Bartlett, Publishers.

United States Congress (August 1986). *The "Black Box" of Home Care Quality.* Report of the Select Committee on Aging, House of Representatives, 99th Cong., 2nd Sess., prepared by the American Bar Association, Committee Publication No. 99–573 U.S.G.P.O.

Watts, D., & McCally, M. (1984). Demography. In C.K. Cassel & J.R. Walsh (Eds.), *Geriatric Medicine* (Vol. 2, pp. 3–15). New York: Springer-Verlag New York, Inc.

Chapter 6

The Regulation and Organization of Home Care

Marshall B. Kapp

Home care providers may be organized, from a legal and financial viewpoint, in a variety of different ways. The legal form that a particular provider takes may influence that provider's regulatory (and common-law [see Chapter 9]) status and obligations.

In terms of ownership, a home care agency may be either (1) *public*; (2) *private not-for-profit*; or (3) *proprietary*. Public agencies are those that are owned and controlled by a unit of government, such as a state or county. Private not-for-profit agencies are those that are owned and operated by a private group, such as a religious, fraternal, or community group, but without stockholders who expect to be paid financial dividends out of profits generated by the agency. These types of agencies are sometimes termed "charitable" or "voluntary."

Proprietary agencies exist for the primary purpose of making a monetary profit; they are owned by stockholders who invest their money in the agency with the expectation of being paid dividends out of the agency's profits. Such agencies are sometimes termed "investor-owned." In practical terms, today the primary significance of the not-for-profit versus proprietary distinction in home care (and in the health care industry generally) lies in determining whether an agency will be considered taxable or tax-exempt by the federal Internal Revenue Service, according to Internal Revenue Code Section 501 (c)(3).

Private, not-for-profit, and proprietary home care agencies may operate either as *independent* providers or as part of a corporate *chain*. In the first situation, the agency usually is incorporated as an entity that exists legally and financially on its own, whereas in the latter a large corporation may own and run several different home care agencies under one organizational and financial umbrella. In addition, home care agencies that are *owned and operated by an acute care hospital* are becoming an increasingly common phenomenon. Such an affiliation may result either from the hospital developing its own home care agency or purchasing an existing one.

Regardless of ownership status, most home care agencies enter into a variety of legal and financial arrangements with other health and human service providers (eg, acute care hospitals, durable medical equipment companies, nursing homes, and employment agencies) pertaining to the recruitment and serving of clients. These arrangements may be informal (unwritten) but more often are formal (written). These arrangements include contracts and subcontracts for services or products, as well as *joint ventures*. Frequently, many different kinds of organizational arrangements exist between a home care agency and other corporations simultaneously.

In a joint venture, a home care agency and another corporation, such as a hospital, agree to work together for the purpose of recruiting and serving home care clients. A joint venture may take the form of a general or limited *partnership* or a *new corporation*.

A home care agency may also have relationships with health maintenance organizations (HMOs). In return for a prospectively paid single premium, an HMO promises to provide comprehensive health care, which in many HMO contracts includes home care, to its members. An HMO may satisfy this obligation either by owning and operating its own home care agency or by contracting with an existing one to provide services to HMO members in return for payments (either based on a capitation or a fee-for-service formula) from the HMO.

A home care agency may also enter into relationships with preferred provider organizations or arrangements (PPOs/PPAs). Although the variety of specific forms it may take is virtually infinite, essentially a PPO/PPA is an agreement by a group of providers to serve a defined group of clients, such as the employees of a large corporation, at a reduced rate in return for the organization with control over that group of clients (eg, a large corporation that provides health care coverage for its employees, retirees, and their dependents) creating economic incentives for members of the client group to use the "preferred" providers. By joining in PPOs/PPAs, a home care agency may, by agreeing to charge reduced rates, secure a defined segment of the potential client market.

A detailed analysis of these different organizational forms and their legal ramifications is beyond the scope of this book. Suffice it to say here that a home care agency should retain competent legal counsel (see Chapter 8) to assist it in considering, negotiating, and executing any arrangements with other provider agencies. Specific questions that agency staff and directors should pose to legal counsel about any contemplated agreement include those relating to the tax implications, resulting locus of organizational control (including managerial control over staff), reimbursement maximization considerations, legal liability exposure (see Chapter 9), and additional regulatory requirements.

REGULATORY ISSUES

There have been allegations that the American home care industry today is largely unregulated, amounting to a legal "black box" (United States Congress, 1986). Despite these complaints, home care agencies and their staffs, regardless of their specific organizational structure, are held legally accountable in most respects under a panoply of federal and state statutes and regulations and the case law that has interpreted them. This section discusses the regulatory environment of home care.

Licensure

Traditionally, licensure of health care providers, both of individuals and organizations, has been a matter of state responsibility. As of early 1989, 39 states plus the District of Columbia require the licensure of home care agencies by the state (Johnson, 1988; Sabatino, 1989). A list of these state statutes and implementing regulations (where present) is appended to this chapter (Appendix 6). Most state licensure statutes closely mimic the federal Medicare conditions of participation regulations (see below) on home care, although several states (especially New York, Delaware, Connecticut, and the District of Columbia) have enacted more stringent provisions. Approximately a dozen of these state statutes currently delineate a Bill of Rights for home care clients.

Since licensure in these 40 jurisdictions is required as the basic permission of government for an agency to conduct home care activities, it is applicable regardless of an agency's source(s) of funding. In addition to their power to force a home care agency to cease activity altogether (that is, to permanently revoke or temporarily suspend a license) in instances of serious violation of important licensure standards, especially when client safety is compromised, many of these states have the authority under their licensure acts to impose intermediate sanctions, such as civil money fines, injunctions, criminal penalties, or conditional licensure.

In addition to these 40 statutes that license the home care agency directly, there exist in every state statutes that regulate individual health care professionals (such as physicians, nurses, psychologists, social workers, and physical and occupational therapists), regardless of their employment setting. The home care agency must ensure that the health care professionals it employs directly or for whose services it contracts possess legally appropriate credentials, including individual professional licensure (a topic discussed further in Chapter 9).

The home care agency must keep abreast of any limitations placed on the permissible service activities of individual health care professionals by state licensure statutes, implementing state regulations (ordinarily published by the state health or social service department), or state attorney general interpretations of state law. For instance, a 1988 California attorney general opinion interpreted state law to provide that an unlicensed home care companion, whether certified by a voluntary professional accrediting body or not, may administer nonprescription drugs but not controlled (under federal and state drug laws) substances to a client in the client's home. The same opinion stated that an unlicensed home care companion, whether certified or not, may not feed a client at home with a nasogastric or a gastrostomy tube (California Attorney General Opinion, 1988).

Certificate of Need Laws

Approximately 30 states today have certificate of need (CON) laws that require state approval—a determination of need (DON)—before the intitiation or expansion of certain home care services. The coverage of these laws varies, but the CON requirement is most likely to be applicable when a home care agency is being started or acquired as a new service offered by a hospital. A DON program requires that certain health care providers prove to a state agency that the services they seek to provide are needed by the community in which they propose to operate; the program is intended to constrict the supply of health care in a geographic area and thereby promote efficiency in service delivery by requiring economies of scale. Violation of the state CON requirement jeopardizes a provider's ability to collect payment for services from public financing programs, mainly Medicare and Medicaid. While the DON process controls an agency's entrance into, or expansion within, the home care marketplace, this process does not involve ongoing monitoring of the quality of services delivered by the agency once those services are on the market.

Medicare Certification

Home care is a covered service under Part A of Medicare, the federal health care financing program for the elderly and the permanently and totally disabled. Medicare, which spent \$2.5 billion for home care in fiscal year 1987, offers coverage that is focused on acute care, particularly periods of recovery following hospital and surgical care. To qualify for Medicare coverage for home care, a need for skilled care must be demonstrated in which the beneficiary must be under the care of a physician, homebound, and in need of intermittent skilled nursing care or physical or speech therapy. Home care aide services are allowable under certain circumstances. On January 1, 1990, Medicare began covering home intravenous drug therapy. Home care benefits are reimbursed on a reasonable cost basis; the beneficiary is exempt from any cost sharing (United States Congress, 1988, p. 4).

To be eligible to receive Medicare payments for services to covered beneficiaries, a home care agency must meet specified requirements enumerated in the federal Medicare statute, United States Code Title 42, Section 1395x (o), and implementing regulations (Conditions of Participation for Medicare Home Health Agencies, 1989). Whether or not an agency is in compliance with federal requirements is determined through inspections conducted by the state-designated Medicare survey agency, usually the state health department (Gray, 1988).

Since the 1980 Omnibus Reconciliation Act (OBRA), Medicare certification has been open to nonprofit and proprietary home care agencies both in states that license such agencies and those states that do not. It has been estimated that out of the more than 14,000 home care provider organizations in the United States today, approximately 5700 are certified to participate in the Medicare program (McCann & Rooney, 1989).

In the OBRA of 1987 (OBRA 87, Public Law 100-203, 1987) printed at *Congressional Record*, Volume 133, No. 205-Part III, December 24, 1987), Congress substantially changed the federal law relating to participation of home care agencies in the Medicare program. Title IV, Subpart B of this statute is entitled "Home Care Quality." Among the most significant provisions of this sweeping new statute are:

1. Under Section 4021, "Conditions of Participation for Home Health Agencies," an extensive list of consumer rights is enumerated. The agency is now required to protect and promote the rights of each individual under its care, including specific provisions relating to:
   (A) The right to be fully informed in advance about the care and treatment to be provided by the agency, to be fully informed in advance of any changes in the care or treatment to be provided by the agency that may affect the individual's well-being, and (except with respect to an individual adjudged mentally incompetent) to participate in planning care and treatment or changes in care or treatment.
   (B) The right to voice grievances with respect to treatment or care that is (or fails to be) furnished, without discrimination or reprisals for voicing grievances.
   (C) The right to confidentiality of clinical records.
   (D) The right to have one's property treated with respect.
   (E) The right to be fully informed orally and in writing (in advance of coming under the agency's care) of:

(i) all items or services furnished by (or under arrangements with) the agency for which payment may be made under Medicare,
(ii) the coverage available for such items and services under Medicare, Medicaid, and any other federal program of which the agency is reasonably aware,
(iii) any charges for items and services not covered under Medicare and any charges the individual may have to pay with respect to items and services furnished by (or under arrangements with) the agency, and
(iv) any changes in the charges or items and services furnished.

(F) The right to be fully informed in writing (in advance of coming under the care of the agency) of the individual's rights and obligations under this law.
(G) The right to be informed of the availability of the new home health agency grievance hotline that this statute now requires each state to establish.

2. Section 4021 (3) for the first time sets strict criteria for qualifications of home health aides, who are the staff members with a predominant role in direct, hands-on contact with the client. Under this provision, the agency must not use as an aide (on a full-time, temporary, per diem, or other basis) any individual who is not a licensed health care professional, unless the individual has successfully completed a training and competency evaluation program that meets minimum federal standards and the individual actually is competent to provide items and services assigned.
3. Section 4021 (a)(6) requires that the home care agency operate and provide services in compliance with all applicable federal, state, and local laws and with accepted professional standards and principles that apply to professionals providing items and services in such an agency.
4. Section 4022 of OBRA 1987 sets forth new requirements relating to state surveys of home care agencies to determine compliance with the Medicare Conditions of Participation. Most notably, this section now requires state survey agencies to conduct such surveys on a surprise, no-prior-notice basis.
5. Section 4023, relating to enforcement, requires the federal Department of Health and Human Services (DHHS) to establish a range of intermediate sanctions, short of dismissal from the Medicare program, that could be imposed on home care agencies found to be out of compliance with specific parts of the Conditions of Participation. These federal intermediate sanctions will include civil money penalties, the suspension of Medicare payments, and temporary receivership.

6. Section 4025 requires the states, as a condition of receiving federal matching funds for their Medicaid programs, to set up for clients receiving services from Medicare- or Medicaid-certified home care agencies a toll-free hotline and investigative unit for complaints about the quality of home care services being received.

Further Congressional changes in both the Conditions of Participation and enforcement mechanisms are likely in the next several years. Regarding the new Conditions of Participation implementing OBRA 87 (Conditions of Participation, 1989), the Health Care Financing Administration is in the process of incorporating more outcome-oriented measures—as opposed to the present structural and process ones—measures into regulatory standards for home care (Lalonde, 1989). "Outcome criteria are used to determine the amount of measurable change resulting from a particular action by the health provider. In actuality, it is often difficult to determine a direct causal relationship between a specific action by the health care provider (such as instruction regarding meal planning, gait training, etc) and measured change in the client's behavior, manifested, for example, by an increase in appetite, the ability to walk from the bedroom to the kitchen, or the mastery of a particular skill" (Haddad, 1987, p. 155). Although there are technical impediments to such an outcome-oriented approach in the home care setting, we are seeing regulatory motion in this direction. Indeed, the need for more, and more definitive, evidence of the linkages between process and outcome has been cited as the most pressing area warranting attention in quality assurance (Lohr, 1988).

In addition, 1987 amendments to the Older Americans Act (Public Law 100-175) authorize demonstration projects aimed at strengthening home care consumer protection mechanisms. Among the possible approaches being demonstrated (Sabatino, 1989, p. 15) are development of a home care ombudsman program analogous to the nursing home ombudsman program (Kapp, 1987, pp. 51–53) and the development of a protection and advocacy (P & A) system for home care similar to the system that is legally mandated for institutionalized mentally ill and developmentally disabled persons. If these demonstrations are successful (a few states, eg, Maine, Virginia, and Wisconsin, already extend ombudsman services to home care), regulatory changes concerning home care consumer protection and corresponding provider obligations may result.

Another regulatory issue tied to Medicare reimbursement for services is utilization review (UR). For a number of years, the necessity and appropriateness (and to a much lesser extent the quality) of institutional health care services has been subject to a UR process, with reimbursement denied for services deemed inappropriate or unnecessary. Federal statutes passed in 1986 require the extension of professional review organization (PRO) review to home care settings. PRO monitoring will take the form primarily of examining readmission of clients to hospitals from Medicare home care and of responding to client complaints about home care quality. A note in the October 20, 1988, edition of *Hospitals* indicated that the Health Care Financing Administration was at that time in the process of negotiating contracts with PROs for home care review.

VOLUNTARY ACCREDITATION

The previous section discussed forms of home care regulation that are public, in the sense of coming from the government (federal or state) and having a mandatory effect on providers (in the case of Medicare certification, at least if the provider wishes to participate in the government financing program). A very important additional source of home care regulation is the process of private, or *voluntary*, accreditation by nongovernmental organizations. While such accreditation is not mandatory (it is often termed a form of self-regulation) in the same way that compliance with governmental regulations is legally required, there may be strong incentives—in terms of prestige, competition for clients and staff, affiliations with other organizations, and in other areas—encouraging home care agencies to achieve voluntary accreditation. The most significant private organization currently involved in accrediting home care programs is the Joint Commission on the Accreditation of Healthcare Organizations located in Chicago (JCAHO) (McCann & Rooney, 1989). In December 1987 the JCAHO Board of Commissioners approved the final version of standards, which were published in 1988 as *Standards for the Accreditation of Home Care* (Joint Commission on the Accreditation of Healthcare Organizations, 1988). The previous Home Care Services chapter has been deleted from the JCAHO's *Accreditation Manual for Hospitals*, and hospital-based home care services are now evaluated according to a tailored survey, using standards identified in Appendix A, Table of Applicable Standards, in the home care manual. Thus, this manual applies to both hospital-based and freestanding home care agencies. The JCAHO's new survey and enforcement program for home care commenced on June 1, 1988, and within the next seven months over 1100 home care agencies had requested applications and 350 were formally reviewed.

The JCAHO's on-site survey process includes an in-depth review of a home care agency's management and delivery of care to individuals in their place of residence. Included in this process are staff and management interviews; home visits and interviews with clients or their caregivers; home care record documentation review; and a review of clinical and administrative policies of the home care agency, including quality assurance activities, governing body bylaws, financial policies and statements, and promotional materials. The following standard and required characteristics from the Patient/Client Care section of the JCAHO *Standards for the Accreditation of Home Care* delineate requirements for client care delivery.

2. Patient/Client Care (PC)

Standard

PC.1 A home care organization admits only patients/clients whose needs can be met by the services it provides.

Required Characteristics

PC.1.1 The home care organization accurately describes the procedures and services it provides.

PC.1.1.1 A statement of the organization's objectives and scope of care or services is distributed to patients/clients, staff, referral and payment sources, and the interested public.

PC.1.1.1.1 The organization's objectives and services are appropriate to the home setting.

PC.1.1.1.2 The stated scope of care or services includes services provided by the organization or through a contractual arrangement.

PC.1.1.1.3 The hours that care or services are available and, if appropriate, the way patients/clients can obtain care or services after office hours are stated.*

PC.1.2 Written admission criteria specify the types of services provided and the patient/client population the services are designed to meet.

PC.1.3 There is a process, defined in written policy and procedure, for:

PC.1.3.1 acceptance of referrals; and

PC.1.3.2 assignment of appropriate staff to conduct a timely assessment of patient/client eligibility for admission.*

PC.1.4 If the patient/client does not meet admission criteria, the referring individual or organization is notified.*

In approximately 26 states, JCAHO accreditation automatically qualifies a home care agency for state licensure. In those states,

---

* The asterisked items are key factors in the accreditation decision process. (Copyright 1989 by the Joint Commission on Accreditation of Healthcare Organizations, Chicago. Reprinted with permission.)

JCAHO inspection reports concerning a particular agency are available to the public under the state's own Freedom of Information Act.

In 1987, the Health Care Financing Administration (HCFA) proposed (*Federal Register*, December 31, 1987) that JCAHO accreditation for home care agencies be afforded the same "deemed" status as is currently enjoyed for hospitals, that is, that an agency that has received JCAHO accreditation be deemed to meet all requirements for Medicare participation, without the necessity of passing a separate Medicare survey. Widespread opposition, including a 1987 American Bar Association resolution, squelched this proposal. However, in 1988, with the advent of its new home care accreditation program, JCAHO reapplied to HCFA for reconsideration of home care Medicare "deemed" status, a proposal that is currently under advisement.

Two other private organizations also engage in aspects of voluntary home care accreditation. Skilled nursing services delivered in the home are accredited by the National League for Nursing (NLN). The National Homecaring Council (NHCC), under the auspices of the Foundation for Home Care, accredits and approves homemaker and home health aide services.

FRAUD AND ABUSE

The fierce economic competition among home care agencies for clients (particularly among agencies affiliated with hospitals) has led to increased government involvement in regulating the business aspects of the home care industry. The most significant legal development in this area was the enactment by Congress in 1977 of the Medicare–Medicaid Antifraud and Abuse Amendments, carrying for their violation a criminal penalty of a $25,000 fine and up to 5 years imprisonment (United States Code, Title 42, Section 1395nn). The main thrust of this legislation was the prohibition of any form of kickback, rebate, or unfair inducement for health care referrals of clients whose care is paid for by the Medicare program. The chief legislative intent was to save the federal government money by eliminating such health care provider practices as double billing for the same service and billing the government for unnecessary services.

In the years following passage of this federal law, few cases were litigated under it. The leading case (*United States v Greber*, 1985) and subsequent interpretations (*United States v Kats*, 1989) gave the statute a very broad interpretation and added to the extensive prevailing confusion about which specific business practices are and are not prohibited as fraud and abuse. Consequently, in the Medicare and Medicaid Patient and Program Protection Act of 1987 (Public Law 100–93),

Congress added two new provisions addressing the antikickback prohibition.

Section 2 of P.L. 100–93 specifically provided new authority to the DHHS's Office of Inspector General (OIG) to exclude a person or entity from participating in the Medicare or Medicaid programs if it is determined that the party is engaged in a prohibited remunerative scheme. This new sanction authority is intended to provide an alternative civil remedy, short of criminal prosecution, that would be a more effective way of regulating abusive business practices than is the case where the only enforcement weapon is a criminal indictment.

In addition, section 14 of Public Law 100-93 required the DHHS OIG to promulgate regulations specifying those payment practices that will *not* be subject to criminal prosecution and that will *not* provide a basis for exclusion from Medicare and Medicaid (ie, those business practices that *will* be considered "*safe harbors*"). This section reflects the generally accepted view that the statutory language forbidding remuneration that induces referrals is so broadly written as to encompass many harmless or efficient arrangements as well.

Accordingly, the DHHS OIG (following a few false starts, see December 23, 1988, and December 28, 1988, issues of the *Federal Register*) published proposed fraud and abuse antikickback regulations in the January 23, 1989, *Federal Register*. These regulations would amend the *Code of Federal Regulations*, Title 42, Chapter 4, Part 1001. These regulations contain specific "safe harbor" provisions concerning the following types of payment practices: investment interest; space rental; equipment rental; personal services or management contracts; sales of practices; referral services; warranties; waiver of deductibles for inpatient hospital care; and discounts, employees, and group purchasing organizations.

A thorough analysis of these provisions is beyond the scope of this chapter. In addition, the reader should be cautioned that at the time this chapter is written, these regulations are at the *proposed* stage, and the final version after public comment and agency modification may contain some changes. In addition, further statutory changes by Congress may be enacted (eg, Congressman Stark's proposed Ethics in Patient Referrals Act, which would prohibit physicians from referring patients to an entity in which the physician has any financial interest, with very few exceptions).

However, some general guidelines for assessing the legality of business practices may be suggested (Hogue, Teplitzky, & Sollins, 1988). Potential fraud and abuse situations of greatest relevance for home care agencies include (1) those in which hospital discharge planners consistently refer most clients to one particular home care agency, despite the existence of other competing agencies; (2) those in which a hospital engages one particular home care agency to perform the hospital's discharge planning function; and (3) those in which there is an agreement for a home care agency to secure valuable materials, equipment, or services at a substantially reduced rate in return for steering clients to particular durable medical equipment (DME) or other companies (Case, 1984). A legal audit to identify and minimize possible fraud and abuse problems should include the following questions.

First, does the proposed business activity comport with common and accepted current practices in the health care field? Is it a reasonable or legitimate business or medical activity under current circumstances? If these questions can be answered in the affirmative, the conduct involved probably is permissible.

Second, does the proposed activity increase the total costs of the Medicare or Medicaid programs? For instance, does the proposed business activity allow the care providers to bill the programs twice for the same episode of treatment? An affirmative answer to this sort of question should give substantial pause to an agency contemplating such activity; indeed, it should motivate a reevaluation of the strategy involved.

Third, is payment for the proposed activity dependent on a percentage arrangement or on the number of Medicare patients served or referred? If so, especially if remuneration ceases when referrals cease, the practice may be interpreted as illegal.

It should also be noted that almost every state has antikickback and antirebate provisions in its own Medicaid statutes (eg, Ohio Revised Code Section 5111.03). For instance, the California Department of Consumer Affairs, in an August 2, 1988, Opinion Letter, "Physician Resales of Pharmacy Services," claims that the California antikickback laws make it illegal for physicians to purchase pharmaceuticals and then resell them at a higher price to their own home care patients. Obviously, every home care agency should be aware of its own state's fraud and abuse provisions, in addition to the federal law.

ANTITRUST

Legal disputes between a home care agency and its economic competitors may arise as a result of various client *steering practices* (Philp, 1985), which are becoming increasingly common in the current era of joint ventures between home care agencies and hospitals and other entities. The home care agency may function as an "upstream provider," that is, one that refers clients from the agency to a particular acute care hospital. Here, however, we are concerned mainly with the agency's role as a "downstream provider," that is, one that receives client referrals from the hospital. In this situation, hospital discharge planners (Arcidiacono, 1988, pp. 144–146) may consistently recommend one specific home care agency, they may explicitly disparage the quality of other agencies, or they may consistently fail to mention the possibility of other available agencies. Similarly, a hospital may restrict participation in its discharge planning process to representatives of only one particular home care agency. In any of these circumstances, potential antitrust issues must be considered (Miles & Philp, 1985).

The primary federal antitrust legislation in the United States is the Sherman Act, United States Code, Title 15, Sections 1–7. This act provides for a sanction of treble damages (three times the actual loss suffered by the injured victim), and contains a number of other potentially pertinent provisions. A legal audit to identify and minimize possible antitrust problems should follow the guidelines given below.

First, if an acute care hospital does not own the home care agency but nonetheless attempts to refer all of its clients to that particular agency, there may be a complaint of "exclusive dealing" in violation of Section 1 of the Sherman Act. Such an arrangement may be documented in an explicit written agreement, but more likely it will be inferred from the circumstances.

Under the "rule-of-reason" type of analysis generally adopted by the courts for antitrust scrutiny in the health care field (*Jefferson Parish Hospital District No. 2 v Hyde*, 1984), inquiry focuses on the actual effect and intent of the questioned practice. Does the arrangement unreasonably restrain trade or competition? The widely used but not legally definitive guideline for assessing the impact is whether the arrangement affects more than 10 percent of the market share of relevant business in that particular geographic area. Is the purpose of an exclusive referral agreement to restrain trade, or is its purpose to enhance competition by creating financial incentives to improve the quality, efficiency, and accessibility of home care services? Do the clients and their families retain the ability to make ultimate choices about their care providers?

There is no "exclusive dealing issue" if a home care agency is wholly owned by the hospital from which it received patient referrals. Two entities that have the same economic interests and are part of the same enterprise by definition cannot conspire with each other to restrain trade.

Tying of Services

If the hospital owns the home care agency to which it steers its discharged clients, the question is one of "tying" of services, which also is covered under Section 1 of the Sherman Act. In this case, the hospital may encourage its discharged clients to use the services of its own home care agency, but it may not legally require such use as a precondition for receiving hospital services. Put differently, the two separate services must be "untied" and available to be purchased by the client either as a package or separately.

In assessing whether outlawed "tying" of services has taken place, the following kinds of questions should be posed: Does the seller, that is, the hospital, have an economic interest in the home care agency? Are all or most of the hospital's clients required to purchase the tied product? Is buying the second product mandatory? Is sale of the hospital care preconditioned on the purchase of home care from a particular (that is, the hospital's) agency? Do the steering tactics go beyond persuasion and recommendation and amount to coercion? Does the client or family retain a meaningful right to choose? When does the steering occur? If the first product, namely acute hospital care, has already been delivered before the steering occurs, there is no tying involved.

Other potential Section 1 violations include price fixing, horizontal market allocation, and group boycott. Price fixing involves an agreement among competitors that has the purpose or effect of fixing or stabilizing the prices at which they sell their services—for example, an agreement between two home care agencies that they will each charge the same amount for their services. Horizontal market allocation involves an arrangement among competitors in which they agree which of them will and will not offer certain goods or services, which of them will and will not compete in certain localities, and which of them will and will not deal with certain clients. If two home care agencies in a locality agree that only one of them will offer medications, while only the other will provide home health aide services, this would constitute an anticompetitive, and therefore illegal, dividing up of the pie.

A group boycott is an agreement among two or more parties not to deal with another party, to deal only on certain terms and conditions, or to prevent a competitor from obtaining a trade relationship that it needs to compete. A group boycott would probably exist, for instance, if home care agencies A and B agreed with a durable medical equipment supplier that the supplier would not deal with new home care agency C in order to hinder agency C's ability to compete in that locality.

Monopolization

A further antitrust issue is monopolization, covered by Section 2 of the Sherman Act. Here, a court would ask whether a hospital has an economic interest in a particular home care agency and, if so, whether the two entities together exercise "monopoly power or control" (roughly, but not definitively stated in law, as more than 60 percent) over either hospital referrals or over the home care market in their geographic area. If "monopoly power" is found, is it the product of willful acquisition, or is it the maintenance of a monopoly for its own sake, which would be impermissible? Are the health care providers engaging in legitimate, procompetitive business practices (trying to increase their own business share by enhancing the quality and efficiency of their services), or are they just engaging in predatory destruction of a competitor?

The antimonopoly statute requires sellers of goods and services to deal with their economic competitors. How far a hospital must go to comply with this provision is unsettled, but it likely means that the hospital must provide competing home care agencies with the same access to clients as is afforded the hospital-affiliated agency (Koska, 1988).

Section 2 of the Sherman Act prohibits attempted monopolies as well as actual ones. For an illegal attempted monopolization to be found, the following elements must be present. First, there must be two separate economic entities. Second, there is as yet no monopoly share (roughly 60 percent of the geographic hospital referral or home care market), but there appears to be a specific intent, inferred from anticompetitive conduct, to achieve a monopoly without legitimate business justification. Third, there must be evidence of a "dangerous probability of success" in capturing a monopoly share of the market. To avoid attempted monopolizations, the law requires sellers to deal fairly with their competitors. In the home care context, that probably means giving competitors an equal opportunity to market their services to prospective clients.

Another related practice outlawed by Section 2 of the Sherman Act is conspiracy to monopolize. A violation of this prohibition entails proof that two or more separate entities specifically and intentionally have conspired or agreed to monopolize the market and have engaged in an overt act in furtherance of the conspiracy (eg, exclusive client referral). This statutory provision heavily overlaps the Section 1 prohibition against exclusive dealing with anticompetitive intent.

In all of the antitrust concerns outlined above, three key analytical factors are involved:

1. What is the hospital's economic importance as a referral source in its community?
2. What is the extent of the home care agency's market power in that community?
3. Are there legitimate procompetitive justifications for the business practices in question?

PRICE DISCRIMINATION

Another potential antitrust-related issue that may be raised by a home care agency's competitors is the allegation of illegal price discrimination. This kind of claim could be brought, for example, where a hospital is able to purchase drugs, DME, or other health-care-related commodities at lower than market prices because of its volume purchasing power and then resells those same items to its own home care agency at reduced, preferential rates (Abood, 1985; Owens & Epstein, 1986). This type of claim could be brought not only against a home care agency that profits directly or indirectly from the preferential pricing of commodity resales, but by a home care agency that is discriminated against by preferential resale practices carried out by others (Miles, 1987).

The federal Robinson-Patman Price Discrimination Act (Public Law 74-692, United States Code, Title 15, Section 13) forbids price discrimination or preference "where the effect of such discrimination may be substantially to lessen competition or tend to create a monopoly in any line of commerce, or to injure, destroy, or prevent competition with any person who either grants or knowingly receives the benefits of such discrimination, or with customers of either of them." There is an exception to this prohibition for nonprofit hospitals (as well as other nonprofit charitable institutions) who make purchases of supplies for the institution's own use. For example, a hospital that offers a reduced price to a former inpatient at discharge for a prescription to complete the therapy begun in the hospital would be operating properly. This exception was created by the Nonprofit Institutions Act (Public Law 75-550, United States Code, Title 15, Section 13C).

The applicability of this "own use" exception to a situation of reduced drug prices for a nonprofit, hospital-based home care agency is presently untested and unclear. At the least, the hospital pharmacy should be intimately involved in consulting with hospital legal counsel before undertaking any sort of business arrangement that involves preferential prices for the hospital's own home care agency (Greenberg, 1986). The pharmacy should maintain comprehensive written records of products sold or given to the home care agency at reduced rates or for free. Also, the hospital attorney should consider conferring with the legal departments of the pharmaceutical manufacturers with whom the hospital transacts business.

This area was complicated further by Congressional enactment in April 1988 of the Prescription Drug Marketing Act. This law contains a broad prohibition against buying, selling, or trading any prescription drug that was purchased by a public or private hospital or that was donated or supplied at a discount to a not-for-profit organization. The problem of product diversion by health care providers is sufficiently bothersome that the Washington (DC) based Health Industry Distributors Association (HIDA) has organized a nationwide network to collect information on suspected illegal resales.

SUMMARY

As the foregoing illustrates, home care agencies are accountable to a panoply of public and private regulators. Standards are set regarding both client care and the agency's business practices, and violation of those standards may expose a home care agency to serious consequences. Devising effective policies and procedures for identifying and complying with applicable governmental standards is vital to a home care agency's legal and fiscal health.

REFERENCES

Abood, R.R. (1985). Differential pricing of pharmaceuticals and retail competition under the Robinson-Patman Act. *American Journal of Law and Medicine, 11*:293–317.

Arcidiacono, K. (1988). Legal aspects of discharge planning. In P.A. O'Hare & M.A. Terry (Eds.), *Discharge Planning: Strategies for Assuring Continuity of Care.* Rockville, Md: Aspen Publishers, Inc.

California Attorney General. (June 15, 1988). *Home Care Companions.* Opinion No. 87–106.

Case, F.H., III. (1984). DME contracting with hospitals. *Caring, 3*(7):27–28.

Conditions of Participation for Medicare Home Care Agencies. (August 14, 1989). *Federal Register*, 54(155), 33354–33373, codified at *Code of Federal Regulations*, Title 42, Part 484.

Gray, J.W. (1988). *Home Health Survey Guide.* Owings Mills, Md: National Health Publishing.

Greenberg, R.B. (1986). Legal implications of home health care by nonprofit hospitals. *American Journal of Hospital Pharmacy, 43*:386–391.

Haddad, A. (1987). *High Tech Home Care: A Practical Guide.* Rockville, Md: Aspen Publishers, Inc.

Health Care Financing Administration. (December 31, 1987). *Federal Register, 52*(251).

Health Care Financing Administration. (January 23, 1989). *Federal Register, 54*(13).

Hogue, E.E., Teplitsky, S.V., & Sollins, H.L. (1988). *Preventing Fraud and Abuse: A Guide for Medicare and Medicaid Providers.* Owings Mills, Md: National Health Publishing.

Jefferson Parish Hospital District No 2 v Hyde, 104 S Ct 1551 (1984).

Johnson, S.H. (1988). Who sets standards for home healthcare? *Health Progress*, 69(11): 20–21.

Joint Commission on Accreditation of Healthcare Organizations. (1988). *Stand-*

ards for the Accreditation of Home Care. Chicago: Joint Commission on Accreditation of Healthcare Organizations.
Kapp, M.B. (1987). *Preventing Malpractice in Long Term Care: Strategies for Risk Management.* New York: Springer Publishing Company.
Koska, M.T. (1988, June 20). Lawsuit prompts CEOs to examine DME ventures. *Hospitals*, p. 86.
Lalonde, B. (1989). Outcome scales for measuring the quality of home healthcare. *Generations, 13*(1):51–53.
Lohr, K.N. (1988). Outcome measurement: Concepts and questions. *Inquiry, 25*(1):37–50.
McCann, B.A., & Rooney, A.L. (1989). The Joint Commission's homecare project. *Generations, 13*(1):54–56.
Miles, J.J. (1987). Commodity resales by nonprofit entities: Antitrust implications for home health agencies. *Caring, 6*(5):64–67.
Miles, J.J., & Philp, M.S. (1985). Hospitals caught in the antitrust net: An overview. *Duquesne Law Review, 24*:489–689.
Omnibus Reconciliation Act of 1987, Public Law 100–203, printed at *Congressional Record, 133*(205) Part III, December 24, 1987.
Owens, J., & Epstein, R.L. (1986). *Legal Implications of Hospital Resales of Pharmaceuticals.* Legal Memorandum No. 7. Chicago: American Hospital Association, Office of the General Counsel.
Philp, M.S. (1985, December 1). Home health referrals: Some legal guidelines. *Hospitals*, pp. 72–75.
Sabatino, C. (1989). Homecare quality. *Generation, 13*(1):12–16.
United States Code Title 42, (1989, August). Medicare Program; *Home Health Agencies: Conditions of Participation*; Department of Health and Human Services.
United States Congress. (1986, August). *The "Black Box" of Home Care Quality.* Report of the Select Committee on Aging, House of Representatives, 99th Cong, 2nd Sess, prepared by the American Bar Association, Committee Publication No. 99-573.
United States Congress. (1988, April). *Home Care at the Crossroads.* Information paper of the Special Committee on Aging, Senate, 100th Cong, 2nd Sess, S Prt 100–102, Serial No. 100–H.
United States v Greber, 760 F 2d 68 (3d Circ), *cert denied*, 474 US 988, 106 S Ct 396 (1985).
United States v Kats, 871F 2d 105 (US Ct App 9th Cir 1989).

Appendix 6. State Licensure Statutes and Regulations for Home Care Agencies

Ariz Rev Stat Sec 36-401 et seq, Ariz Admin Comp R9-10-1101 et seq
Cal Health & Safety Code Sec. 1725 et seq, Cal Adm Code Tit 22, Sec 74600 et seq
Conn Gen Stat Sec 19a-490 et seq, Conn Agencies Regs Sec 19-13-D66 et seq

Del Code Ann Tit 16, Sec 122(3)(h)
DC Code Ann Sec. 32-1301 et seq
Fla Sta Sec 400.461 et seq, Fla Admin Code Sec. 10D-68.001 et seq
Ga Code Sec 31-7-150 et seq, Ga Admin Comp ch 290-5-38
Hawaii Rev Stat Sec 321-11, 321-18, Hawaii Admin Rules Sec 11-91-1 et seq
Idaho Code Sec 39-1301 et seq, Idaho Admin Regs Tit 2, ch 5
Ill Ann Stat ch 111 1/2, Sec 2801 et seq, Ill Admin Code Tit 77, Sec 245
Kan Stat Ann Sec 65-5101 et seq, Kan Admin Regs Sec 28-51-100 et seq
Ky Rev Stat Sec. 216B, 902 Ky Admin Regs 20:081
La Rev Stat Ann Sec 40:2009.31 et seq
Me Rev Stat Ann Tit 22, Sec 2141 et seq
Md Health-Gen Code Ann Sec. 19-401 et seq, Md Admin Code Tit 10, Sec 10.07.10
Mo Ann Stat Sec 197.400 et seq
Mont Code Ann Sec. 50-5-101 et seq, Mont Admin R Sub-ch 3, rule 16.32.307 et seq
Nev Rev Stat Sec 449.001 et seq, Nev Admin Code Sec 449.010 et seq
NH Rev Stat Ann Sec 151.1 et seq, NH Admin Code ch. He-P 809
NJ Stat Ann Sec 26:1A-1 et seq
NM Stat Ann Sec 24-1-1 et seq
NY Public Health Law Sec 3600 et seq, NY Admin Code Tit 10, Sec 765–767
NC Gen Stat Sec 131g-135 et seq, NC Admin Code Sub-ch eL
ND Cent Code Sec 23-17.3-01 et seq, ND Admin Code Sec. 33-03-10
Or Rev Stat Sec 443, Or Admin R ch 333, div. 27
Pa Stat Ann Tit 35, Sec. 448.801 et seq
RI Gen Laws Sec 23-17-1 et seq, R23-17-HHA
SC Code Ann Sec 44-69-10 et seq, Dept of Health & Env Control Reg. No. 61-77
Tenn Code Ann Sec 53-1301 et seq, Tenn Admin Comp ch 1200-8-8
Tex Civ Stat Ann, art 4447u, Tex Admin Comp 115.1 et seq
Utah Code Ann Sec 26-21-1 et seq
Va Code Sec 32.1-162.7 et seq
Wash Rev Code ch 70.126, Wash Admin Code ch 248-27
Wis Stat Sec 141.15, Wis Admin Code ch. HSS 133

Chapter 7

The Employer–Employee Relationship

Amy Marie Haddad
Marshall B. Kapp

Most of this book has been dedicated to the exploration of the ethical and legal obligations of the home care provider to the client and to society at large. This chapter emphasizes another relationship that is integral to the healthy, successful functioning of a home care agency—namely, that between employer and employee. Though there are numerous levels of personnel in a home care agency, the ethics section of this chapter will focus on the relationship between home care management and the homemaker or home health aide. Its legal section will focus on malpractice liability issues that are applicable to all levels of employees in a home care agency.

HOMEMAKER–HOME HEALTH AIDE

Though paraprofessionals in home care provide two distinct types of services, health and housekeeping, the term "home health aide" will be used to refer to all paraprofessionals in the home. The home health aide is an essential and often overlooked and underrated member of the home care team. It is important to explore how the aide is treated in the home and within the agency hierarchy because of the relative powerlessness of the position. By examining how home health aides are treated in comparison to other members of the home care team, we can determine if and how the ethical principles of respect for persons, beneficence, and especially justice are applied in daily practice.

Obviously, not everyone in a home care agency can be treated the same. There are legitimate differences in roles, rights, and duties. But the distribution of burdens and benefits should be accomplished fairly. John Rawls's theory of justice addresses the issue of fair distribution and argues for attempting to maximize the position of those who are minimally advantaged (Rawls, 1971). In the case of the home care agency hierarchy, the home health aide is the least advantaged in terms of salary, educational opportunities, and frequently in the area of fringe benefits.

Rawls acknowledges that inequalities exist, but he would arrange them so that, ideally, inequalities would benefit all affected or at least those most in need. For example, suppose a home care agency limits the number of consecutive hours that staff is allowed to work on extended hour cases. Although this rule works against those who want to work longer, the standard can be justified by showing how such a rule works to the advantage of all concerned—those who do not want to work overtime, the clients (who are the most vulnerable), and even those who want to work more hours, as they will not be permitted to jeopardize their own health and well-being. The key point in this example is that inequalities can only be tolerated when they work to everyone's advantage. Even those who are limited by the inequality must really benefit from it.

A common example of inequality in home care is the practice of rewarding long-term, valued employees by assigning them the "easy" cases and giving the difficult cases to new employees. The employer sometimes rationalizes this practice by viewing it as a test of the commitment of the new employee.

> Such assignments are understandable in an industry where flat pay scales and undifferentiated tasks offer few opportunities to reward deserving workers. The effect of this perverse reward system, however, is to exacerbate turnover among new workers, who are already the most vulnerable to turnover, and to subject the neediest clients to the least experienced aides. (Feldman, 1989, p. 29)

Another example of an inequality that does not work to everyone's advantage is the practice of treating home health aides as independent contractors as opposed to salaried or hourly employees with full benefits. This practice offers the home health aide cash but no minimum benefits such as worker's compensation and unemployment insurance. Though this might be a fair practice with professionals, who can afford to purchase needed benefits on their own, the home health aide is generally not in a financial position to do so. According to Rawls's theory, neither of these examples of inequality is permissible.

HOME CARE PERSONNEL SHORTAGE

One issue that clearly affects all levels of the home care industry is the shortage of competent health care workers. The shortage has reached crisis proportions in nursing.

> The current shortage results from the demand for nurses outstripping the supply. First, medical technology has developed rapidly in recent decades and is increasingly used to treat severely ill patients. Second, the number of such patients has increased because of both the aging of the population and medicine's success in keeping patients alive longer. Third, the number of new nursing graduates has decreased due to the expansion of career opportunities. (Roberts, Minnick, Ginzberg, & Curran, 1989, p. 2)

The shortage differs from city to city but is much more evident in urban areas. The majority of nurses are still employed in hospitals (approximately 63 percent). Home care providers used to be able to attract nurses who wanted a change from the acute care setting. With the overall decrease in the number of available nurses, there will be a concomitant decrease in the number of nurses interested in making the change to home care.

The shortage of home health aides is equally severe. Among the reasons for the shortage of home health aides is the increased need for long-term care services such as basic hygiene, feeding, dressing, meal preparation, chore services, and light housekeeping. The primary consumers of these types of services are the frail elderly and the chronically ill. As the number of frail elderly increases, so does the need for paraprofessional supportive care. In addition, competing industries, such as national cleaning services and fast-food restaurants, are siphoning off potential homemaker–home health aide workers by offering better wages and fringe benefits ("Improved H–HHA Image," 1989, p. 2).

The shortage puts additional demands on the existing home care staff as well. The charge facing the home care industry is to keep well-qualified employees and to attract sufficient workers to fill the ever-growing need for staff. However, selling the job of home health aide is getting more difficult all the time. A study found most of New York City's 70,000 home care workers to be minority women. A third of them made less than $5000 per year (many are not full-time employees). The same study noted that 48 percent of all home care agencies reported severe recruitment problems for home health aides, and 37 percent also reported severe retention problems (Koska, 1988). If wages and fringe benefits are not what they should be, are working conditions any better? What type of person is attracted to home care? What type of people does the industry want? Are the responsibilites of the job commensurate with the satisfactions?

The home health care industry could not exist without home health aides, yet the job still holds a less than positive image. Facing all of these issues is a painful but necessary step toward survival in a competitive market for competent, caring employees.

MORALE AND JOB SATISFACTION

Are home health aides born or made? Either way, there are certain character traits and skills that are desirable in a home health aide. Morally good habits or character traits are also known as virtues. Since the overwhelming majority of home health aides are women, the virtues of a home health aide can generally be defined in terms of the stereotypical roles of wife and mother. Therefore, a home health aide is expected to be nurturing, compassionate, sensitive, patient, courageous, and self-sacrificing. They are also expected to be technically competent within their sphere of responsibility which includes, minimally, the following tasks: personal care, physical activities, environmental tasks, and social and emotional support.

A similar discussion regarding the standard of qualifications for nurses is documented in Isabel Hampton Robb's book *Nursing Ethics: For Hospital and Private Use*, which was published in 1901. Though the discussion centers around nurses, it is equally applicable to the qualifications of a home health aide.

> Those of us who have had much experience in nursing, and know all we would have a nurse to be, and how much she really must be, as the various classes of women pass in review before our mental vision, will be inclined to agree with the writer of a letter which came to me sometime since. After asking me to recommend a head-nurse for a hospital, and enumerating at length the qualities she must possess to be successful, he concluded with the words, "In short, we require an intelligent saint." (Robb, 1901, pp. 39–40)

It is not realistic to expect home health aides to be saints but are the expectations of the role realistic? This leads us back to the initial question with some modification—are good home health aides born or made? It is clear that not everyone wants to work in home health care. So those individuals who express interest in home care are in a sense bringing the raw materials to the home care employer. Fortunately, we do not have to rely on heredity to provide the makings of a "good" home health aide. Virtues are learned and practiced; they can be taught. Therefore, if the home health employer expects specific virtues and duties of their home health aides, it is the employer's obligation to provide the training and support necessary to fulfill these expectations. Besides technical training, the home health aide should receive instruction in human value areas such as confidentiality, client rights, and the extent of their obligations to clients and families (Aalberts, 1989).

Attention must be given to the sort of work environment necessary to make these virtues flourish in the context of home care. The role of the home health aide in the home and in the home care organization will be explored next in order to cite ethical pitfalls and to suggest what the home care employer can do to prevent or resolve these problems.

The Home Health Aide's Role in the Home

Home health aides, as well as other home care providers, are often unclear about their specific role in the home. This uncertainty is compounded for the home health aide because of a proliferation of titles that refer to paraprofessional services depending on the specific funding sources involved. If the home health aide is vague about his or her role, entering the home setting will probably not help clarify it.

Health care institutions are, more or less, neutral territory. Health care workers in an institution are clearly in charge and dictate, among other things, schedules, activities, and visitation privileges to name a few. The home care setting provides far fewer guidelines for role definition. The home health aide and other caregivers are "guests" in the home and at the same time are delivering care and services to clients and their families. If the home health aide provides physical care and some light housekeeping tasks such as meal preparation, the role of the home health aide may become further confused with that of "servant" or "maid." Role confusion may be accentuated by the cultural mix of clients and staff, which is often more obvious in home care than in institutional care.

To resolve the natural confusion about the role of the home health aide in the home, the home care employer must emphasize the duties of the home health aide in standardized training programs, which now have been incorporated in the Conditions of Participation for Home Care Agencies implementing the Omnibus Reconciliation Act of 1987 (United States Code Title 42, Section 1891(a)(3)(D)) (see Chapter 6). These nationally mandated training standards will educate home health aides, who have the most contact with the client and who were, prior to the enactment of these standards, often poorly prepared for their responsibilities (Hodges, 1989).

In addition, the home care agency, usually through the nursing supervisor who oversees the work of the home health aide, should plan carefully for the staff's presence in the home before instituting service. The client and family need to be briefed in detail regarding the extent of the duties of the home health aide so they do not place the home health aide in the awkward position of refusing to do requested tasks that are outside of their job description.

Another problem that relates to the role of home health aides is the endemic isolation in which they work and the lack of surveillance of their work. Home health aides generally work in isolation from their coworkers and supervisors. "The opportunities for validation and clarification are limited. The informal exchanges between staff members that allow for ventilation and support are missing" (Haddad, 1987, p. 131). There is a strong sense of loneliness on the part of most home health aides that can contribute to burnout. The supervision of home health aides is generally done at a distance.

> Most supervision of homemaker–home health aides is carried out by case coordinators (schedulers) who spend most of their time in the office, much of their day on the telephone, and who rarely visit the aide in the home. Substantive decisions about the care of the client are usually made by the agency nurse. In contrast to the coordinator, the nurse spends much of her time in the field. However, in many agencies, her case load is so large that she may visit a given home only three or four times a year. (Feldman, 1989, p. 29)

Without adequate training and education, the home health aide can only draw on life experiences to help resolve the problems encountered in home care. The home health aide needs more than maturity to resolve the problems encountered in home care, a problem that lends even more support to the need for standardized training. In addition, a new type of field staff, such as a senior home health aide, has been suggested to help support the home health aide and diminish feelings of isolation. The senior home health aide could visit the home on a more frequent basis than the nursing supervisor and work on a team basis with the home health aide and others assigned to the case. The new field staff could provide support, report back to the home care agency on the progress of the case, the home health aide's performance, problems encountered, and the need for additional training (Feldman, 1989). Currently, there are no reimbursement sources for this type of support field staff.

Specific Ethical Difficulties for the Home Health Aide

The majority of the ethical issues cited throughout this book apply to the home health aide as well as the agency itself. However, there are several issues that appear to be more problematic because of the job description of home health aides, their level of preparation, and their place within the organizational structure.

The Noncompliant Client. The home health aide, who often has little training or hands-on experience, ends up spending a great deal of time relatively independently with a very sick or chronically ill person. When this very sick person will not cooperate, the home health aide's job becomes more difficult, if not impossible. When a client doesn't comply with the proposed plan of care, he or she is often regarded with a great deal of frustration and labeled as "noncompliant." Generally, when a client will not cooperate with the plan of care, a reason is sought. The home health aide may easily exhaust his or her abilities to discern the cause of the noncompliance and choose to follow one of two paths, neither of which is ethically desirable.

First, the home health aide may use coercion to force the client or family to comply with the treatment plan. In its extreme, this coercion may take the form of physical force or verbal threats. Second, the home health aide may resort to falsifying clinical records and other documentation such as travel logs in order to make it appear that the care has been delivered as ordered when, in fact, it has not.

Training and support are needed to help the home health aide deal with difficult situations such as the noncompliant client. The home health aide must realize that frustration alone is never a sufficient reason for coercing the client, falsifying records, or neglecting care entirely. The home health aide should be encouraged to discuss his or her anger and frustration with the immediate supervisor when confronted with a difficult client or family member.

There are, however, situations in which the home health aide would be justified in withdrawing from a case, such as in the instance of potential or threatened violence. In determining whether aides should be expected to take personal risks in caring for potentially violent clients home care management should consider that: (1) personal sacrifice is required only when there is some possibility that something beneficial may be achieved by it; and (2) it is both prudent and morally acceptable to take steps to protect oneself (Jameton, 1983). In cases of potential violence, home health aides should remove themselves from harm and immediately report the situation to the home care agency.

Moral Distress. Moral dilemmas are conflicts in rights and responsibilities that call for a choice between unappealing alternatives.

> Most moral dilemmas present a need to balance competing ideal claims in untidy circumstances. The reasons on each side of many moral problems are weighty, and none is obviously the right set of reasons. Indeed, there is a sense in which all the reasons ought to be acted on, for each, considered by itself, is a good reason (Beauchamp & Walters, 1982, p. 4).

For example, the commitment of a family to care for a chronically ill child at home may lead parents to provide care past the point of emotional and physical exhaustion, yet obligations to the other children in the family may lead the parents to consider institutionalization of the ill child. Both alternatives are unappealing, yet each places claims upon the parents that cannot be ignored.

More often, individuals are involved in less dramatic ethical decisions. Rather than being caught between two or more unappealing alternatives, the individual is drawn to a choice but cannot act on it, a situation that results in moral distress. "Moral distress arises when one knows the right thing to do, but institutional constraints make it nearly impossible to pursue the right course of action" (Jameton, 1984, p. 6). The home health aide's role is complex, requires considerable responsibility, and yet has limited authority. These factors place the home health aide in the middle of many ethical conflicts in the home as the following case study shows.

Case 7–1. Reporting Suspected Abuse

Mary Ellen Borg, 78 years old, lives with her 76-year-old husband, Fred, in the one-bedroom apartment they have occupied for 30 years in one of the older housing redevelopments in a large urban center. Mary Ellen has Parkinson's disease, which has resulted in contractures, an extremely unsteady gait, and a constant tremor that makes eating and self-care almost impossible. Fred is an alcoholic who has been sober for the last eight years but suffers the consequences of years of alcohol abuse; cirrhosis, congestive heart failure, and lapses of memory. Fred is able to take care of himself and the house, but not Mary Ellen. A neighbor suggests that the Borgs call the local visiting nurse association to get some assistance with Mary Ellen's care. Finances are limited and the nursing supervisor who receives Fred's call suspects that the Borgs might be eligible for Medicaid.

In addition to a speech therapist, skilled nursing visits, and a social service worker, a home health aide named Louanne Fuller is assigned to assist Mary Ellen with her personal hygiene, ambulation, and feeding twice a week. Fred has been taught how to get Mary Ellen up and to dress and feed her. Fred is able to complete these care tasks successfully in the nurse's presence. However, after the first week, Louanne is certain that Fred is not taking care of Mary Ellen as well as he should. Mary Ellen is soiled and agitated when Louanne arrives. Mary Ellen is also thirsty and hungry, appears malnourished, and is losing weight. Louanne asks Fred if he is having any difficulties in caring for Mary Ellen. Fred replies, "She's awful heavy. I get her up when I can. I ain't no nurse, you know. Besides, I think she could do more if she tried."

On her next visit, Louanne notices that in addition to being dirty and hungry, Mary Ellen is bruised on the left side of her face and her right elbow is bruised and abraised. When Louanne asks Mary Ellen how this happened, Mary Ellen merely shakes her head. Fred appears uninterested when Louanne asks him about the injury and says, "Why don't you ask her? She can talk good if she wants to."

Louanne suspects that Fred is abusing or, at the very least, neglecting Mary Ellen. Though other members of the home care team are involved in Mary Ellen's care, Louanne sees her most frequently and has become quite fond of her. Louanne has seen this type of situation before. She knows what happens when cases of suspected or obvious abuse are reported to adult protective social services. Louanne is certain that if she reports her suspicions to the proper authorities, this action will destroy whatever trust the Borgs have in her. She is almost as certain that, even if she reports the case, nothing will be done. The caseworkers for adult protective services are overloaded and many times are unable to resolve a situation like this one. Finally, Louanne can identify with Fred's frustration. Mary Ellen is difficult to take care of and doesn't always cooperate. At this point, although Louanne knows the "right" thing to do—report suspected abuse to her supervisor—she perceives bureaucratic constraints that discourage her from pursuing the right course of action.

Though Louanne is probably correct in thinking that she cannot "change the system," she can work with her peers to identify those aspects of Mary Ellen's care that can be changed. Also, some of the moral distress that Louanne feels can be mitigated by the various strategies suggested throughout this chapter, such as standardized training and more support from colleagues and supervisors in the field. Home care administrators ". . . need to provide more opportunities for staff to attend outside meetings and conferences [regarding elder abuse]. These are not merely educational, but are important ways for health care providers to increase morale through informal sharing of experiences" (DeRenzo, 1989, p. 12). Instruction in bioethics, through in-service education, can also play a part by encouraging home health aides to express themselves more confidently regarding the ethical issues they encounter.

Conflicts Between Coworkers. Though there are changes on the horizon to make the role of the home health aide more attractive, there is still considerable confusion and devaluation of the role. When a group is devalued by society, self-hatred or hatred of one's own group is the result. In home care, when home health aides are devalued, they often turn their anger and frustration against members of their own group. This aggression against one's own group has been termed "horizontal hostility" or violence against one's own peers (Kennedy, 1970). Horizontal hostility becomes manifest in the home care setting in the form of sibling rivalry and competitive dueling. If home health aides do not receive psychologically necessary approval from their supervisors or employer, they will seek it from the family and the client. When the goal is the approval of the family and the client, home health aides can become rivals and may work against rather than with each other. This rivalry often takes the form of undermining the work of colleagues. The infighting evident in the following case study is every supervisor's nightmare.

Case 7–2. Infighting Among Staff

Nancy Kokorda and Mary Jo Peters had both been assigned to Mr. Benedict's case. Mr. Benedict was the victim of an automobile accident. He sustained a closed-head injury that severely hampered speech, bowel and bladder control, and ambulation. The legal settlement from the accident provided Mr. Benedict with twenty-four-hour coverage for home health aides on an indefinite basis. Nancy had been assigned to the case when Mr. Benedict came home from the hospital. She worked with the nursing supervisor to establish a plan of care to include a daily schedule of personal care—a bath, oral hygiene, changing linen—and a program to encourage bowel and bladder continence. Mary Jo was assigned to the evening shift on the case approximately 1 month after Mr. Benedict returned home.

As far as Nancy was concerned, Mary Jo could not do anything right. Nancy used the "message book" that was supposed to help with communication between shifts to air her grievances regarding Mary Jo's performance. The supervisor could not discern any obvious differences between the two aides' work. Both treated Mr. Benedict with care and concern. Both complied with the standard of care established by the agency. Yet, Nancy was not satisfied. The supervisor knew that the stakes in this game of one-upsmanship had escalated when Mrs. Benedict called to complain about Mary Jo's care. Mrs. Benedict wanted Mary Jo removed from the case. Though Mrs. Benedict could not give any specific reason, she just wasn't happy with Mary Jo's work. With further probing, Mrs. Benedict admitted that she really hadn't noticed a problem until Nancy brought it to her attention.

This scapegoating of one home health aide by another typifies the broader issue of aggression against the group. Usually something is at stake: approval (of the family or home care administrator) or some other gain (to be completely in charge of a case). The home health aide's self-esteem, however, is the real underlying issue. In this case, it was as if Nancy could only be up by putting Mary Jo down.

The passive–aggressive behavior evidenced in this case has ethical implications on three levels. First of all, there is the potential for psychological harm to the client and the family. The trust that is at the heart of the relationship between the caregivers and the client and family is threatened. Second, there is potential harm to the coworker who is the target of the undermining behavior. For example, if true improvement or change is needed, the only effective way to bring about this change is through direct communication. By talking behind people's backs and then acting surprised when they somehow find out, we are doing a double disservice—we are not fulfilling our obligation to do good and we are not showing respect. Finally, there is direct harm to the home care agency by diminishing its reputation with the client, family, and the community at large.

To resolve the conflict between Nancy and Mary Jo, the home care supervisor has to model the behavior she or he wishes to see in the home health aides. Therefore, the supervisor must be active rather than passive in discussing the situation with Nancy and Mary Jo. The supervisor must be certain that there is no real need for concern regarding Mary Jo's abilities to deliver safe, responsible care. If Nancy has informally been given the responsibility to "manage" Mr. Benedict's care, she should also be given additional training to help her effectively coordinate his care. Home care managers have acknowledged this need for status and distinction on the part of their more experienced home health aides and have established in-service programs to fulfill those needs. For example, "aides who have at least three years of experience may be sent to a 'Supervision in Home Care' seminar, offered annually, after which they may participate, under professional supervision, in some aspects of case and service management" (Feldman, 1989, p. 44).

RESOLUTIONS

All of the resolutions suggested so far have one thing in common—that home health aides are worthy of the same respect as other members of the home care team. Home care supervisors and managers should extend the same respect to their staff that they themselves expect to receive. Therefore, staff should be given appropriate assignments with adequate training to perform their jobs safely and effectively.

The input of home health aides should be actively solicited regarding the care of the clients in their case loads. Involvement of the home health aide in the decision-making process should begin in the training phase of employment. This behavior can then be reinforced by involving home health aides in decision making and problem solving in team meetings or client staffings, thus expanding their knowledge of the total home care process (Tuttle, 1989). Initially, it may be difficult to convince home health aides that their input is valuable. This may be evidenced in low attendance at conferences and in-service sessions. To remedy this and to recognize the value of their time, it is appropriate to pay home health aides for the time they spend in conferences and in-service programs.

Another way of providing recognition for performance and experience is through career advancement strategies, such as credentialing programs, which have positive effects on employee motivation, job satisfaction, and staff retention.

A credentialing program is a formally established system for developing, evaluating, and promoting individuals within an organization. The home health agency should initially identify a system of recognition and reward that is consistent with the agency's organizational structure, goals, and present performance appraisal system. The credentialing program must include performance criteria that are incrementally staged to reflect more responsibilities. The new federally mandated training standards could serve as the basis of a credentialing program. Each home health aide must meet these basic training requirements. The home care agency could then build upon this base with in-service education and specific types of experiences that would constitute the criteria for advancement to a higher level of functioning, perhaps designated by a different title such as "senior home health aide" or "home health aide II," which is rewarded with increases in pay.

This type of career advancement program, whether for home health aides or professional staff, requires a commitment of resources on the part of the home care agency. Therefore, even though there are significant positive outcomes from career advancement programs, these benefits must be balanced against the economic welfare of the agency as a whole. Home care managers are challenged to provide career advancement opportunities in response to severe shortages of personnel, yet be equally responsive to the need for agency productivity and cost-conscious management.

Regardless of financial constraints, the home care agency must structure an environment that is humane and fair to all of its employees. It is more costly, in every sense of the word, to treat employees as a means to an end. Employee mistreatment is neither ethical nor practical in this environment of competition and scarcity of valuable personnel.

MALPRACTICE ISSUES

In addition to the ethical implications of the home care agency's role as an employer of personnel, this role also raises a number of legal issues, especially concerning malpractice liability issues. In the home care context, the agency and its staff may be forced to defend against claims predicated on theories of personal, vicarious, or corporate liability. The remainder of this chapter explores these three theories of liability and offers illustrations of their application to the home care setting.

Personal Liability

Personal liability is the doctrine that holds an individual responsible for what he or she personally does or fails to do. Each of us may be held legally answerable for our personal acts or omissions. Thus, for example, a physician who prescribes the wrong drug or dosage for a client may be held personally liable for that error, assuming that it directly caused injury. Similarly, the nurse who administers the incorrect drug or dosage without adequately questioning or checking on the order's accuracy may be found personally responsible for that negligent omission.

In reviewing the legal theories that may expose parties *beyond* personal liability, it must be remembered that the potential presence of vicarious or corporate liability in no way eliminates the possible personal liability of any parties for wrongful personal conduct. Put differently, vicarious or corporate responsibility may be imposed in addition to or on top of, and not in place of, a negligent party's personal liability.

Vicarious Liability

In addition to claims that may arise from an individual's personal conduct, the staff member's supervisors and the home care agency itself may also face vicarious liability for the individual's misconduct. Under the principles of "agency," a "master" (employer, supervisor, principal) is civilly liable for injuries to the person or property of third persons caused by the negligence of a "servant" (employee, supervisee, agent) that occurred within the scope of that servant's employment or job responsibilities. The idea of "scope of employment" for vicarious liability purposes has been interpreted quite broadly by the courts.

This version of vicarious liability is known as the *respondeat superior* doctrine.

Respondeat superior also applies to intentional as well as negligent wrongdoing of the subordinate, but only in those situations in which the superior should reasonably have foreseen the intentional misdeed. If an employee harms a client by intentional, even criminal acts, such as assault and battery (abuse), theft from a client, or breaking and entering a client's home without permission, those acts may expose the home care agency to possible civil or monetary liability if a jury can be convinced that the agency should have been able to predict and control the employee's behavior (Gould, Ginsberg, & Perdew, 1986).

Given the proper factual predicate, the same vicarious liability principles that relate to paid agency employees may also be applied to the use of volunteers, students who have been placed with the agency as part of a learning experience, and private companies that act as the home care agency's agent. In this regard, the key is identifying whether an individual or company is functioning in a particular situation as agent of the home care agency or as an independent contractor. The chief question is whether the home care agency had the legal authority to control and direct the subordinate, both in terms of final result and the specific methods for achieving that result. An affirmative answer to this question would indicate a principal–agent relationship entailing potential vicarious liability for the home care agency.

If the home care agency only hired a professional or company to achieve a particular result (such as installation of a specific piece of equipment in a client's home) but did not retain the authority to direct the particular method and details of installation, the hired individual or company would be acting as an independent contractor. In that situation, the home care agency would not be exposed to vicarious liability for the independent contractor's negligence. Other potential liability considerations, though, are involved in the use of independent contractors, and these considerations are discussed in Chapter 9. The status of someone as an employee or as an independent contractor is not necessarily dependent on the intention of the parties or on how the parties themselves characterize their relationship, although those factors may shed light on the ultimate determinative question of control (Gilliland, 1988).

It should also be noted that, in addition to vicarious liability concerns, characterizing the relationship between a home care agency and an individual as either one of employment or independent contracting makes an important difference for purposes of: Social Security (FICA) retirement payments; income tax (see *Internal Revenue Service Bulletin* 1987-41 and *IRS Technical Advisory Memorandum (TAM)*

8749001); the Fair Labor *Standards Act* (FLSA) and its provisions for minimum wages and overtime pay; unemployment compensation; antidiscrimination provisions of Title VII, Civil Rights act of 1964, 42 United States Code Sec 20003; and compliance with federal immigration laws (Gilliland, 1988). Home care agencies should develop and regularly apply self-review criteria to keep straight the legal status of their relationships with individuals with whom they conduct business activities.

There are also several negligence doctrines that have been cited to expand the reach of *respondeat superior*, such as "borrowed servant," "shared servant," and "captain of the ship." Since these doctrines have mainly been used to expand physician liability in the institutional environment, this chapter does not elaborate on them (although theoretically they might be applied to physician supervision responsibilities in the home care setting).

Several arguments traditionally have been proposed to justify the imposition of liability upon an employer or supervisor who is personally innocent of misconduct. *Respondeat superior* is often defended as a form of enterprise liability, in which the business entity that profits from the activity of a subordinate is more justly considered the risk taker or loss bearer. Also frequently cited is the "deep pocket" theory, which asserts that an injured person should have the right to seek compensation from an economically solvent defendant, who is more likely to be the employer than the employee. In addition, the employer is in a better position than the employee to approximate future damages and to treat them as an operating expense. In other words, an employer is able to purchase liability insurance coverage to guard against the contingency of being held vicariously liable for the employee's negligent actions. Further, since the "master" has the power to select its "agents" and to control their job-related behavior, the *respondeat superior* doctrine would seem to promote the desirable social policy of encouraging greater care in the selection of subordinates and in the supervision of their work.

These policy rationales logically apply to the home care industry, as does an additional one. In the home care area especially, the client usually entrusts total personal welfare to a specific agency and its professional staff, and it is that provider and those individual staff members who have accepted that trust and who should bear the burden of ultimate responsibility for the quality of care delivered.

Respondeat superior, although no-fault from the supervisor's and agency's vantage point, is not exclusively a form of strict or absolute liability, since some substandard conduct by a subordinate must be present in order to hold the supervisor or agency liable. Specifically, a supervising health care professional or agency may not be held legally liable for the misdeeds of a subordinate unless a jury finds as a matter of fact that the subordinate gave negligent care that directly caused a client to suffer financially compensable injuries.

STAFF SUPERVISION AND VICARIOUS LIABILITY

Effective control of legal risks dictates that the home care agency, as an employer and therefore a principal, must properly supervise the activities of its employees and agents. With regard to staff, the agency assumes a legal duty to carefully hire and adequately train, supervise, and monitor performance. This obligation extends to both professional and nonprofessional employees, as long as they perform tasks that in any way impact on client welfare. Likewise, appropriate care in the selection, training, and oversight of the agency's volunteers and students is equally important.

Carrying out this responsibility properly, particularly where adverse actions such as discipline or termination must be taken concerning specific staff members, is frequently a tough assignment. There are financial and pragmatic considerations, such as the shortage of qualified, conscientious personnel who are clamoring to work in home care, that may impair the sort of staff selection and supervision that seems most ideal legally and clinically. Problems in recruiting, monitoring, and maintaining decent personnel, especially at the level of the nursing aide, who usually has the most extensive personal contact with the client, have been well-publicized (United States Congress, 1988). Sometimes compromises must be made. However, economic and demographic factors like the relevant local labor supply at a particular moment will not be successful as a defense to a claim imposing vicarious liability on a home care agency for the errors and omissions of its staff. From a legal perspective, which focuses essentially on the client's welfare, staffing difficulties "come with the territory" of home care ownership and management and correction lies within the agency's turf.

Similarly, federal and state labor laws may make it more difficult for the agency to easily select and reward good staff and to discipline or terminate unsatisfactory staff, especially in situations where parts of the staff are unionized or threatening unionization. Despite any limitations imposed on employers by the labor laws, the home care agency's responsibility to fulfill its supervisory role regarding its staff remains undiminished. The laws protecting employees from arbitrary and capricious treatment by employers will not prevent a home care agency that acts with sufficient foresight, planning, fairness, deliberation, and documentation from controlling staff activity that may threaten clients, other staff, or the agency (Gould, Ginsberg, & Perdew, 1986). Agency contracts with employees and employee unions must be negotiated from the perspective of avoiding lawsuits by clients as well as avoiding grievances by employees (Perdew, 1986).

Every home care agency should carefully and regularly examine its relationships and agreements with staff, volunteers, educational programs, and independent contractors. This audit should cover policies and procedures as well as substantive content, and it should be done with an eye toward managing legal risks associated with selection, training, and monitoring responsibilities. At the least, the following suggestions (which build and elaborate on home care Management and Administration Standards 6 through 8 of the Joint Commission on Accreditation of Healthcare Organizations [JCAHO]) (Joint Commission, 1988, pp. 27–28) should be considered:

1. The job titles and performance of all staff and volunteers associated with the home care agency should be reviewed periodically. The development of written job descriptions that are shared with the individuals involved often will clarify lines of authority.
2. To ensure that each individual provider meets basic professional standards, at the recruitment phase the agency must have evidence that each employee has the appropriate legal credential for the practice of his or her profession (eg, nursing, social work, physical, occupational, and speech therapy, pharmacy). In addition, the agency must be able to assure clients that the professionals involved in their care possess current basic and specialized knowledge necessary to fulfill their duties (Perdew, 1986). It is the agency's obligation to match the job assignments and activities for each employee with that employee's level of credentialing, knowledge, and ability, and to ensure that assignments do not exceed the employee's legal and professional capacity to perform.
3. The agency should have a means for continually evaluating the performance of all staff and volunteers and for correcting inadequate performance. This process should overlap with, draw on, and contribute to the agency's overall risk management system (see Chapter 9).
4. The agency should develop and periodically update a policies and procedures manual detailing the functions to be performed and the expectations and standards demanded of all staff, volunteers, and students.
5. A thorough professional development program for orienting and training and retraining staff and volunteers to maintain professional competency and morale should be developed and implemented (Gould, Ginsberg, & Perdew, 1986; Jernigan, 1987).
6. Where the agency is involved in teaching programs that entail

the placement of students within the agency in contact with clients, credentials of supervising faculty members must be assessed and documented (Perdew, 1986) and clear supervisory responsibilities must be negotiated and recorded explicitly.

LIABILITY OF INDIVIDUAL PROFESSIONALS FOR NONSUPERVISION

As noted in the earlier discussion of *respondeat superior*, although the home care agency itself may face possible vicarious liability for failure to properly monitor and supervise staff, individual staff members may also be held legally responsible for the acts or omissions of other employees, volunteers, and students where a supervisor–supervisee relationship exists. Thus, for instance, an agency nursing or social work director may be held vicariously liable, even though he or she did nothing wrong personally, for the wrongdoing of subordinates who are assigned to function under that director's ultimate supervision and control. The key is not the actual degree of control exercised, but whether the supervisor had the authority and the responsibility to direct the nature and the specifics of the subordinate's performance if the supervisor had chosen to exercise such control. The obvious lesson is that supervisory duties must be discharged with great seriousness.

One area of home care participation and supervision that has so far been quiescent redundant, but that is potentially explosive legally, is that of physician involvement. In 1965, when Congress originally included home care among the reimbursable Medicare services, it sought to shore up physician involvement in home care by conditioning the agency's reimbursement on the physician (acting either as an employee of the agency or as an independent contractor) authorizing and supervising the home care treatment plan. (In addition, Medicare Conditions of Participation require that the policies of certified agencies be "established by a group of professional personnel . . . including one or more physicians. . .," 42 Code of Federal Regulations Sec. 405.1201 [a].) Despite this nominal requirement of physician participation, however, the actual record of meaningful physician involvement in home care services is mediocre at best, with the physician's signature often representing little more than a tacit accommodation to permit third-party reimbursement of the agency (Koren, 1986; United States General Accounting Office, 1981).

The failure of many physicians to take seriously their home care responsibilities represents a legal minefield. We agree with the assessment that

> Although lawsuits on behalf of patients receiving home care have been few in the past, it would be unrealistic to expect this situation

> to continue. As doctors prescribe home care for patients discharged from hospitals, they will become increasingly responsible for ensuring that their orders and services are correctly and professionally implemented. (Koren, 1986)

In addition to being exposed under the vicarious liability theory for failure to supervise others in the medical aspects of a client's home care, a physician also runs the risk of personal liability for deviating from acceptable professional standards in rendering home care services (Atkinson, 1987). First, the physician–client relationship does not terminate merely because a client's care shifts in location from a hospital to the home. If the client continues to need direct or supervised medical services (which is the case in virtually all home care situations), and the physician–client relationship that existed in the hospital has not formally been terminated by notice to the client and a reasonable attempt to refer the client to another competent physician, the physician retains the duty of care inherent in the physician–client relationship when the client is discharged from the hospital to the home. Failure to follow through on that duty, if injury to the client results, constitutes the tort of *abandonment*, exposing the physician (and possibly the home care agency that failed to properly monitor physician activity) to substantial monetary damages.

For the physician who follows the client from the hospital into the home or who accepts a referral and begins to see the client in the home after hospital discharge, medical performance must meet "accepted practice" standards (not merely satisfy "customary practice") requiring conformity with medical practices that have been approved by the medical community at large (King, 1975). Such "accepted" medical practice would be exemplified by the American Medical Association's endorsement of active physician participation in its official 1987 home care policy statement and by the standards for physician supervision contained in Medicare regulations (42 Code of Federal Regulations Sec. 1223). Courts generally find this kind of evidence persuasive, and deviation from "accepted" practice so defined would constitute legally actionable negligence.

Hence, we join strongly with those who advocate much more conscientious physician involvement in home care. Further information may be obtained from the American Academy of Home Care Physicians, P.O. Box 924331, Houston, Texas 77292–4331.

CORPORATE LIABILITY

Vicarious liability is called a *derivative* form of liability, because it derives from and depends on the relationship between the party in the superior position and the subordinate who was personally at fault. In addition to legal exposure under the vicarious liability doctrine, a home care agency may also be held legally liable to a client *directly*, that is, based on its own independent relationship to the client. A home care agency's own direct liability to an injured client rests on the theory of *corporate liability*. In the context of an actual lawsuit, the doctrines of vicarious liability and corporate liability, although analytically distinct, are often both relied on in the plaintiff's complaint.

A home care agency's potential corporate liability raises a number of important implications. In terms of procedure, the ability to sue the facility directly may enable an injured client to succeed even where the available evidence would not support a finding of vicarious liability. In addition, suing the agency on a direct liability theory may provide the plaintiff with a longer statute of limitations than the vicarious liability theory would support.

From a substantive viewpoint, the corporate liability theory imposes on a home care agency a variety of specific duties. These duties include:

1. The duty to properly purchase and maintain, or to properly recommend and monitor the purchase and use of, equipment, supplies, medication, and food.
2. The duty to develop and implement appropriate written institutional policies regarding client safety.
3. The duty to screen, train, monitor, and supervise agency employees, volunteers, and students carefully.
4. The duty to carefully screen, monitor, and supervise independent contractors with whom the home care agency has a business relationship (see Chapter 9).

OSTENSIBLE OR APPARENT AGENCY

A further source of potential home care agency liability should be mentioned here. Where circumstances make it reasonably apparent (ie, make it seem) to a client or a client's family that a physician or other provider is functioning as an agent or employee of a home care company (even though in fact the provider is an independent contractor for whose errors the home care agency otherwise would not be held legally responsible), any negligence by that provider may be imputed to the home care company under the legal doctrine of *apparent or ostensible agency*. The sort of circumstance that might activate this doctrine would be if the home care agency were to assign a private physician to a client when the client's former physician is not willing to continue the client's care in the home. In that situation, the client might claim that she or he reasonably believed that the physician was an agent of the home care company and accordingly relied on that belief in placing trust and confidence in that physician. Where appearances that are within a provider's control create reasonable beliefs that in turn foster detrimental client reliance, the courts may use the apparent or ostensible agency doctrine as a matter of fairness and treat the appearance as though it were the reality.

In addition, the common law (judge-made law) of apparent or ostensible agency may be expanded by current industry standards requiring home care agencies to monitor the quality of care delivered by independent contractors. Those monitoring duties are discussed in Chapter 9.

EMPLOYEE SAFETY

The preceding section of this chapter has explained some of the potential liability concerns of a home care agency based on the acts or omissions of employees that result in injuries to clients. It must be remembered that a home care agency also owes certain duties to its own employees, volunteers, and students to protect them against predictable injuries that may occur in the course of their activities on behalf of the agency. Employees face the risk, for example, of being involved in car accidents while traveling to or from a client's home, being victimized by crime (either in the neighborhood of a client's home or by the client or client's family), straining themselves while lifting the client or a heavy object, slipping and falling in the client's home, being sexually harassed by a client or fellow worker, or contracting a contagious disease (the emergence of the AIDS epidemic raising a particularly frightening if unlikely example) from a client or household member (Orlikoff & Vanagunas, 1988). In a service-intensive enterprise such as home care, legal claims by employees hold a significant possibility for the agency to experience financial loss (Gould, Ginsberg, & Perdew, 1986).

Ordinarily, the Workers' Compensation insurance that the home care agency is legally required to carry will provide financial compensation to an employee (or volunteer or student functioning in the equivalent capacity of an employee) for job-related injuries. The status of independent contractors in this regard is a matter still unclear in labor law. Other forms of insurance carried by the home care agency as a corporation, such as automobile liability, property, or casualty coverage, may also be applicable to employee accidents. To keep its Workers' Compensation and other insurance premiums under control, each home care agency should devise and regularly review policies and procedures designed to minimize foreseeable, preventable injury risks to employees, should train employees to minimize risks in accordance with agency policies and procedures, and should include information and strategies about employee injuries in the agency's overall risk management program (Chapter 9). Any legal action filed by an employee against the agency should be handled through, or at least communicated to, the agency's designated risk management officer.

REFERENCES

Aalberts, N. (1989). Training home care paraprofessionals: Areas for consideration. *Caring, 8*(2):26–27.

Atkinson, S.C. (1987). Note, Medicare 'cost containment' and home health care: Potential liability for physicians and hospitals. *Georgia Law Review, 21*:901–927.

Beauchamp, T.L., & Walters, L. (1982). *Contemporary Issues in Bioethics* (2nd ed.). Belmont, Calif: Wadsworth Publishing Company.

DeRenzo, E.G. (1989). Elder abuse: Ethical theory in everyday practice. *Caring, 8*(3):10–12.

Feldman, P.H. (1989). The Ford home care project: Reducing turnover among paraprofessionals. *Caring, 8*(2):28–29.

Gilliland, J.C., II (1988). Employees versus independent contractors. *Caring, 7*(9):58–64.

Gould, E.J., Ginsberg, A., & Perdew, S.R. (1986). Home care challenge. *Caring, 5*(9):74–83.

Haddad, A. (1987). *High Tech Home Care: A Practical Guide.* Rockville, Md: Aspen Publishers Inc.

Hodges, J. (1989). A national cerification system for paraprofessionals: A report of a grant-funded training project. *Caring, 8*(2):32–33.

Improved H–HHA image needed to address increasing shortages. (1989, February). *Homecare News*, pp. 1–2.

Jameton, A. (1983). Making hard choices. In S. Gorovitz, R. Macklin, A.L. Jameton, J.M. O'Connor, & S. Sherwin (Eds.), *Moral Problems in Medicine* (2nd ed.) (pp. 126–137). Englewood Cliffs, NJ: Prentice-Hall, Inc.

Jameton A. (1984). *Nusing Practice: The Ethical Issues.* Englewood Cliffs, NJ: Prentice-Hall, Inc.

Jernigan, D.K. (1987). Managing risk in the home health setting. *Home Care Economics, 1*(2):46–52.

Joint Commission on Accreditation of Healthcare Organizations. (1988). *Standards for Accreditation of Home Care.* Chicago: Joint Commission on Accreditation of Healthcare Organizations.

Kennedy, F. (1970). Institutionalized oppression vs the female. In R. Morgan (Ed.), *Sisterhood Is Powerful* (pp. 438–446). New York: Vintage Books.

King, J. (1975). In search of a standard of care of the medical profession: The 'accepted practice' formula. *Vanderbilt Law Review*, 28:1213–1276.

Koren, M.J. (1986). Home care—who cares? *New England Journal of Medicine, 314*:917–920.

Koska, M.T. (1988). Aides shortage limits home health delivery. *Hospitals, 62*(9):63.

Orlikoff, J.E., & Vanagunas, A.M. (1988). *Malpractice Prevention and Liability Control for Hospitals.* Chicago: American Hospital Publishing, Inc.

Perdew, S.R. (1986). Litigation in home care: What the future holds. *Caring, 5*(9):84–88.

Rawls, J. (1971). *A Theory of Justice.* Cambridge Mass: Harvard University Press.

Robb, I.H. (1901). *Nursing Ethics: For Hospital and Private Use.* Cleveland: J.B. Savage.

Roberts, M., Minnick, A., Ginzberg, E., & Curran, C. (1989). *What to Do About the Nursing Shortage.* New York: Commonwealth Fund.

Tuttle, D. (1989). The impact on quality: Homemaker–home health aide training. *Caring, 8*(2):41–44.

United States Code Title 42. (1989, August). Medicare Program; *Home Health Agencies: Conditions of Participation*; Department of Health and Human Services.

United States Congress. (1988, April). *Home Care at the Crossroads.* Information Paper of the Special Committee on Aging, Senate, 100th Cong, 2nd Sess, S Prt 100–102, Serial No. 100–H.

United States General Accounting Office. (1981). *Medicare Home Health Services: A Difficult Program to Control* (HRD–81–155). Washington, DC: US Government Printing Office.

Chapter 8

The Role of Legal Counsel in Home Care

Marshall B. Kapp

Home care providers, like other entrepreneurs—both proprietary and nonprofit—frequently regard getting good legal advice as a time-consuming hassle, but failing to obtain the services of an able lawyer in a timely fashion can be a serious mistake (Tannenbaum, 1989).

Though health care practice seems overly concerned with avoiding malpractice litigation, many businesses and agencies, including those in the health services area, operate with next to no legal counsel. Some seek to save money, at least in the short run, or they want to protect their privacy or to maintain total control over enterprises they consider personal. Others think lawyers raise all sorts of hypothetical problems, increase the cost of doing business, and make it difficult or impossible for the agency to achieve its dual objectives of client service and financial viability. In addition, a naive tendency to underestimate legal risks and implications often characterizes health care professionals, even in today's highly regulated environment.

WHEN TO USE LEGAL COUNSEL

The first rule of employing legal counsel is common sense: if home care personnel *think* that they need legal advice regarding a particular matter, they probably do—for purposes of maintaining peace of mind, if nothing else. It is wiser to err on the side of seeking legal advice and being counseled that there are no serious legal impediments to the home care provider's proposed course of action than to proceed without legal guidance and discover at a later point in time that there are legal problems that have arisen.

Another general guideline is that, since potential legal liabilities arise out of breaches or violations of duties, and since duties arise out of relationships formed between two or more parties, legal counsel is advisable whenever a relationship is being formed between two or more parties or an important transaction is occurring as part of such a relationship. Thus, for instance, all contracts for the purchase or sale of goods or services, employment agreements, leases, covenants, or other documents involving the home care agency in a formal relationship with other entities or individuals ought to be reviewed by legal counsel. Certainly, any business relationship such as a corporate purchase or sale or joint ventureship of the agency requires legal involvement. Agency operating policies and procedures, while they may appear at first blush to be matters of internal concern only, affect the reasonable expectations of—and therefore the home care agency's legally enforceable relationships with—staff and clients (and their families), and therefore command legal attention in their drafting, revision, and application. Of course, any litigation involving the agency either as a plaintiff (the complaining party in lawsuit) or a defendant (the responding or answering party) in a court or administrative tribunal calls for legal counsel. Regulatory activities, which define the relationship between the agency and government, are also a matter of legal concern.

Many of the preceding examples illustrate rather obvious situations where legal counsel is imperative. A home care agency's retention of and reliance on its attorney(s) should not be restricted to such obvious examples. Input of legal counsel ought to be integrated fully on an ongoing basis into the whole range of agency service and management activities. A good lawyer should be used by the agency not only to perform strictly "legal" duties, but in addition to act as a more general sounding board and all-purpose advisor.

The home care agency must understand that its attorney is one part of a larger consultative team of professionals that the agency can call upon for advice and representation in planning, initiating, implementing, monitoring, and defending its various activities. While a good attorney ought to be capable of performing a wide array of functions, the home care agency must have a realistic set of expectations concerning both the abilities and the limitations of legal counsel. The availability of a competent attorney will not eliminate the necessity for the agency to retain other professionals such as accountants, realtors, and management and labor consultants for particular projects. Legal counsel should be involved on a regular basis in interacting with the other members of the professional consultative team acting on behalf of the home care agency.

Selection of Legal Counsel

In selecting legal counsel, the home care agency should begin by identifying the purpose or purposes for which legal counsel is being considered. The practice of law today is every bit as specialized an enterprise as is the practice of medicine. The attorney who is best qualified to represent the agency in an antitrust or fraud and abuse matter may not be the same attorney that the agency should retain to handle labor issues.

The attorney best suited to negotiate a joint ventureship or contracts with vendors rarely will be the home care agency's ideal choice for implementing a risk-management program designed to reduce legal risks associated with clinical services or for representing the agency in litigation. In short, while a home care agency should consider hiring in-house legal counsel or retaining one law firm to oversee its legal affairs generally, it is unlikely that any but the very largest single firms would possess internally all the legal expertise involved in handling effectively the broad range of legal needs confronting the modern home care agency. Thus, under the umbrella of a general oversight law firm or in-house counsel, a home care agency should anticipate the probability of hiring several different law firms over the course of time to work on different aspects of the agency's business.

For home care agencies seeking to hire an attorney, choosing one can seem a daunting task; the United States has an estimated 660,000 lawyers, with the number growing exponentially by the year. There is a strong temptation to turn for an attorney to a tennis partner, a relative, or the telephone book. While these techniques on occasion may lead to satisfactory results, the odds run in the opposite direction.

Some better alternative modes of selection exist. First, there is no substitute for the recommendations, based on personal experience, of other home care agencies regarding a particular law firm. Satisfied clients are the best advertisement for an attorney (or any other professional or firm). National and state associations to which home care agencies or their staff members belong may be able to supply recommendations.

Most local bar associations operate lawyer referral services. These programs rarely screen firms on their referral list beyond checking state licensure and membership in the local bar association, and they usually provide a list of three or four firms without making a specific recommendation or endorsement. Nonetheless, this process can be a useful starting point for an agency's further investigation concerning the particular expertise and experience of a firm.

There are several professional organizations in the United States today to which attorneys specializing in branches of the health law field may belong. Although these associations ordinarily do not operate lawyer referral services, a home care agency should inquire of a prospective law firm whether its members belong to and are involved in the activities of such organizations. Major organizations in the health law field (and their headquarters location) include: the American Society of Law and Medicine (Boston); the National Health Lawyers Association (Washington, DC); the American College of Legal Medicine (Chicago); and the American Academy of Hospital Attorneys (Chicago).

National specialty board certification does not exist in the legal profession in any way comparable to the system found in medicine. Several states (for example, Florida), though, have adopted modified forms of specialty designation for attorneys. A home care agency should check with its own state bar association to ascertain whether a lawyer specialty designation system exists in that jurisdiction and, if so, what designations are available. Prospective attorneys may then be questioned concerning their own designation status.

A very useful aid in acquiring information about particular attorneys is the Martindale–Hubbell publication. This is a multivolume reference work, updated annually, that can be found in virtually any law library and almost all decent-sized public libraries. It contains basic biographical and educational data concerning every licensed attorney in this country. In addition, law firms that purchase display listings provide valuable information about representative clients, specialties, and publications and professional accomplishments of their members.

It should be borne in mind that the home care agency will not always maintain control over the selection of its legal counsel. In the case of litigation in which the agency is sued as a defendant, the agency's legal counsel ordinarily will be selected and paid for by the agency's liability insurer, as a benefit spelled out in the agency's insurance policy. While the attorney in that circumstance works in effect for the insurance company, generally the insurance company has a financial interest that dictates the provision of competent and vigorous legal defense on behalf of the agency.

Retaining a Law Firm

In other situations, where the home care agency has both the authority and the responsibility to choose (and pay for) legal counsel, the agency should not be too intimidated or reluctant to interview several law firms to whom the search has been narrowed. Retaining a law firm is like a marriage in many ways, and the agency should feel comfortable with a law firm's particular expertise, experience, reputation, and—extremely important—style and personality, before slipping the retainer ring on its finger.

Home care agencies also should not be bashful about comparing and negotiating professional fees with law firms with whom they are engaging in a courtship ritual. Fees should always be discussed and agreed upon explicitly and before the agency has formally entered into a relationship with the firm; agency management should raise the topic early if the attorney does not.

Law firms are businesses, which must sell their services within an increasingly competitive economic marketplace. Most firms will quote new prospective clients a standard fee structure, usually based upon an hourly rate; most law firms charge at different rates for the time of partners (shareholders or owners of the firm) versus associates (attorney employees of the firm), paralegals, and investigators. Some law firms charge an integrated hourly rate, meaning that the client will be charged the same fee regardless of which particular individual(s) in the firm actually expended the time on the client's behalf. A small but growing number of law firms now accept clients on a prepaid basis, in which the client pays an agreed-upon amount to the law firm at the beginning of a specified time period in return for a designated package of legal services, regardless of the actual time it takes the law firm to provide those services.

Whichever rate schedule is quoted to the home care agency by a law firm, a couple of points must be kept in mind. First, the agency should insist on clarification both initially and on a periodic basis of which specific individuals within a law firm will actually be doing the work on the agency's account. For many legal needs of the agency, the services of a law firm's senior partner are not essential, and having the bulk of the work performed by junior partners, associates, or paralegals (functioning under attorney supervision) makes good sense. Nonetheless, the home care agency has the right and the duty to know what it is paying for and receiving in terms of legal services.

Second, the professional fees quoted by law firms to prospective clients, even when introduced as the firm's "standard" rate structure, are not necessarily etched in stone. The home care provider, as a possible large client with an extensive and ongoing portfolio of legal work to be delivered to a law firm, may be in a position to bargain and negotiate preferred rates with law firms, in the same manner that large corporations today create or bargain with preferred provider organizations (PPOs) of health care entities for the discounted provision of health services to the corporation's covered beneficiaries.

Once a home care agency has selected, negotiated fees with, and formally retained one or more law firms to act on its behalf, the agency should cooperate fully with the law firm in terms of providing all requested information and documents and paying bills promptly. Interaction and communication with the law firm should be carried out on a continuous, two-direction basis. It is in the agency's interest to comply in a timely and courteous fashion with instructions and requests of the law firm.

At the same time, the home care agency should carefully and continually monitor the performance of the law firm or firms that it retains. Responsibility for this monitoring function ought to be fixed with a particular individual within the agency (eg, in-house counsel, risk manager, quality assurance coordinator, administrator). Large agencies may wish to explore the retention of one of an increasing number of private companies that specialize in monitoring and auditing the quality of legal services provided to health care corporations. Any questions, problems, or dissatisfactions regarding legal services should be reported promptly to the law firm; most complaints by clients about attorneys boil down to instances of faulty communication and are easily solvable.

When the agency's unease or dissatisfaction with its law firm's response to the client's needs cannot be alleviated, the option of transferring to a different firm should be exercised. One of the other reasons, besides the need for specialized professional expertise and experience, that a home care agency should consider spreading its legal business over several law firms is to prevent the agency from becoming excessively dependent upon, and consequently captive to, any one particular firm. The awareness of competition can serve as an effective deterrent to a law firm's complacency and taking the client for granted.

SUMMARY

For a variety of reasons, the modern home care agency requires legal services on a regular basis. Unfortunately, securing and taking advantage of such services can be an intimidating and anxiety-ridden process for most health care providers. The matter of legal representation for home care agencies is influenced by a panoply of important individual factors. The particular history, needs, and resources of the agency, the legal climate of the jurisdiction, and the availability of law firms in the geographic vicinity with requisite competencies in different relevant subject areas will affect the selection, retention, compensation, and monitoring of legal counsel.

This chapter offers a few general guidelines that must be applied to the specific situation of each agency. The consistent watchword, though, is that the home care agency should think of itself as a consumer that is entitled to and should not be hesitant to bargain for and demand high quality, fully accountable legal services at a reasonable and known price.

REFERENCE

Tannenbaum, J.A. (1989, February 15). Small-business owners must pick a lawyer judiciously. *Wall Street Journal*, p. B2.

Chapter 9

Legal Liability to Clients

Amy Marie Haddad
Marshall B. Kapp

Case 9–1. The Malfunctioning Ventilator
Case 9–2. Unrealistic Expectations of Home Care
Case 9–3. A Question of Abandonment

Relatively few lawsuits have been filed to date by, or on behalf of clients against home care agencies. This low-risk experience, however, should not lull home care providers into a false state of complacency.

INFLUENCING FACTORS REGARDING LITIGATION

The following social, economic, and technical factors are emerging and combining to make litigation initiated by or for clients a much more important aspect of home care concern in the coming years:

- Complex technology
- Personnel challenges
- Consumer expectations
- Cost-containment pressures

Complex Technology

For one thing, as the technology associated with home care becomes increasingly complex, the opportunities for things to go disastrously wrong grow as well. Technologically dependent children accepted for home care, who can demonstrate large amounts of future lost earnings as a result of technology-connected mistakes or failures, create a new pool of especially potent potential plaintiffs (Perdew, 1986).

Personnel Challenges

Second, unique personnel challenges increase the possible liability exposure of home care agencies. As the variety and number of personnel required by home care agencies rapidly expand, so too expands the reliance by home care agencies on independent contractors (see below) to satisfy their staffing demands. In addition, the diffusion of home care services throughout a wide array of sites and delivery by a wide array of individuals present special management information and supervision difficulties for home care agencies, which can make it more problematic to control legal risks.

Consumer Expectations

Third, as competition for home care consumers heats up within the health care industry, the likelihood increases that explicit and implicit promises will be made to consumers, through agency advertising or other agency or consumer contact. The expectations of consumers and their families are becoming more demanding, and they are increasingly willing to hold home care agencies accountable to those expectations. Furthermore, there is a growing public perception that every home care agency is part of a wealthy industrial conglomerate, for whom paying legal damages would not be an unfair burden (Gould, Ginsberg, & Perdew, 1986).

Cost-Containment Pressures

Fourth, current cost-containment pressures in health care carry the potential for a proliferation of client-initiated litigation in home care. With public (ie, Medicare and Medicaid) reimbursement tight and private insurance for home care still relatively underdeveloped, a substantial proportion of home care expenses are being paid out of the client's or family's own pocket. Understandably, clients and families are eager to receive what they perceive to be their money's worth and are increasingly aggressive in registering complaints (including complaints in the form of litigation) when they believe the value of services received falls short of their expectations.

In addition, prospective payment systems (PPS) and other current cost-containment mechanisms are reducing the incidence and length of hospital stays significantly and correspondingly inceasing the need for postacute forms of care. Consumers and their families who are upset at what they believe to be premature hospital discharge may well be tempted to act out their frustrations by bringing lawsuits against the home care agencies that take over care for the discharged client.

For these and other reasons (such as the sheer growth in the number of older persons needing home care services, the growth in the number of home care agencies, and the proliferation of governmental and private organization policies and standards for home care), potential legal liability to clients is a subject that should command the careful attention of home care agencies and staff (American Hospital Association, 1987). The remainder of this chapter outlines particular areas of risk, defenses, and risk-management strategies.

CONTRACTS WITH CLIENTS

One source of potential liability of home care agencies to clients is based on breach or violation of contract. This may occur under several legal theories.

Advertising

The agency may be held to have made express or implied promises to clients in the form of claims made about quality or price of services contained in the agency's advertising or marketing materials. Promises placed in brochures distributed to the public, for instance, may be introduced in evidence to establish that an agency undertook a specific duty. Hence, the exercise of prudence in marketing efforts (even—or maybe especially—in this age of competition) is imperative, unless the agency is ready to be held accountable for every claim made in, or reasonably inferred from, its marketing materials.

Service Contracts

A home care agency may also be held liable for failure to fulfull promises made directly to clients (or their surrogates), either orally or in the form of written admission and service contracts. Such written contracts should be drafted carefully, with the assistance of knowledgeable legal counsel, and explained fully to the prospective client (or surrogate), using this document as an opportunity for meaningful client education (Jernigan, 1987). The admission and service contract should specifically set forth:

1. Provider's and client's respective roles and responsibilities.
2. The length, type, frequency, and limitation of services.
3. Costs and payment schedules.
4. Provisions for informed client or surrogate consent for specific interventions on both an initial and a continuing basis (see Chapter 3).

The guiding principle must be avoidance of any promise whose carrying out the agency cannot control or for whose violation the agency is not willing to be held answerable.

Promises to Other Providers

Another possible source of contractual liability stems from promises made by home care agencies to other providers about the client. As one author (O'Neil, 1988) has explained this theory, suppose that a contract exists between a hospital and a home care agency for continuity of care of clients, and that the contract contains an agency promise to the hospital that clients will be assessed for home care services within twelve hours after notice of hospital discharge. Even if the client or surrogate had no direct knowledge of this contractual promise, the agency deviating from its promise—its self-imposed duty—might be held legally liable to the client (as third-party beneficiary of the hospital–home care agency contract) for damages resulting from the failure to fulfill that promise. Thus, enforceable duties both to other providers and to clients who are intended to benefit from the home care agency's relationship with other providers compels care and deliberation in the drafting of promises between agencies and others.

NEGLIGENCE

The possibility of tort liability for professional negligence or malpractice (that is, for unintentional errors or omissions leading to the occurrence of foreseeable and preventable injuries) looms as an important legal mechanism for controlling the quality of services delivered by a home care agency to its clients and for compensating clients who are injured as a result of the agency's professional malpractice. In order for a plaintiff–client to succeed on a negligence claim against a home care agency, each of four essential elements must be proven by a preponderance of the evidence:

1. A duty owed, defined by the applicable standard of care.
2. A breach or violation of that duty.
3. Injury or damage.
4. A proximate or direct causation link between the violation of duty and the resulting injury.

Once a home care agency undertakes the care of a client, the agency is under a duty to perform that care in a reasonable manner (Atkinson, 1987). As the level of home care becomes more sophisticated, the responsibility of providers increases because the standard of care rises to reflect the improving state of the art of acceptable practice. In determining the appropriate standard of care for the reasonable or prudent provider, judges and juries typically seek guidance from one or more of the following sources of evidence (Johnson, 1988; O'Neil, 1987):

1. *Expert witnesses* who are qualified by education and experience to shed light on the relevant issues through testimony about, among other things, the current standard practice in the field.
2. *Federal and state government regulations* setting forth public expectations about appropriate provider conduct. In some jurisdictions, violation of governmental requirements establishes *negligence per se,* that is, proof *by itself* that negligence has

occurred. In other jurisdictions, governmental requirements count as one, but only one, piece of evidence on the legal standard of care for tort liability purposes, to be considered along with other evidentiary sources, such as the present industry consensus or standard practice.

3. *Voluntary standards* of private, nongovernmental professional or trade organizations, such as the Joint Commission on the Accreditation of Healthcare Organizations (JCAHO) (Joint Commission, 1988; *Darling v Charleston Community Memorial Hospital*, 1965), the National League of Nursing, and the National Association for Home Care. In *Darling v Charleston Community Memorial Hospital*, for example, the Illinois Supreme Court found a hospital negligent based on, among other factors, the hospital's failure to comply with JCAHO standards (at the time). The court used the voluntary standard to create a presumption of what the legal standard should be.
4. *Internal policies and procedures* of the home care agency, under which clients have a reasonable expectation of being treated.

Under the personal, vicarious, and corporate liability theories discussed in Chapter 7, a home care agency and its staff may be exposed to liability for negligence of clients. Since the agency performs, or fails to perform, its functions through the actions (or inactions) of its staff, the area of selection, monitoring, and supervision of professional and paraprofessional staff represents one of the major liability danger zones in home care. An important recent national survey of quality issues in home care found that the most frequently cited complaint was lack of appropriate agency supervision of staff, particularly of home health aides (Applebaum & Christianson, 1988). Although the importance of appropriate agency activity in this realm is discussed in Chapter 7, we reemphasize it here as well.

SUPERVISION OF STAFF

The courts have held home health agencies liable for deficiencies in training, credentialing, supervising, and allocating responsibility among staff members (*Roach v Kelly Health Care*, 1987). In the *Roach* case, the court relied on the Oregon home care licensure statute as persuasive evidence of the acceptable standard of care. Although control over staff may be more difficult in the geographically dispersed home care situation than in an institutional environment, standards of care ordinarily are not relaxed to reflect the practical logistical challenges (Greenberg, 1986).

The agency's responsibilities regarding staff screening, supervision, monitoring, and assignment (including reassignment if necessary) are imposed by common-law tort principles, state licensure statutes (*Roach*), and federal Medicare law (Title 42, *Code of Federal Regulations* Section 405.1220). In addition, home health standards of JCAHO bear directly on this subject (Joint Commission, 1988). Pertinent JCAHO provisions include those that require the agency to ensure that:

8. Home Health Services (HH)
Standard
HH.1 The number, qualifications, and current competence of the individual(s) providing each service are appropriate to the patient or client needs, the skills necessary for the level of care required, and to applicable law or regulation.

Required Characteristics
HH.1.1 Each individual who provides home health services has a current license, registration, or certification, in accordance with applicable law or regulation.
HH.1.2 For each home health service, written criteria state the minimum education, training, and experience required for individuals who provide service.

Standard
HH.2 The number, qualifications, and current competence of the individuals supervising home health staff are appropriate to the scope of home health services provided.

Required Characteristics
HH.2.1 Appropriate supervision is available during all hours services are provided.
HH.2.2 All home health services have ongoing supervision.
HH.2.2.1 When a supervisor does not have appropriate clinical training and experience for a clinical specialty area, the organization provides access to qualified consultation.

The Personal Care and Support Services (SS) chapter of the Joint Commission home care manual contains an extensive list of standards for staff training and supervision for organizations that provide personal care or other support services (eg, assistance in activities of daily living, maintenance and management of household routines).

These services may be provided directly or through contract with other organizations.

In sum, a home care agency must do at least the following (Kapp, 1987):

1. Properly screen staff, both for legal authority (eg, professional licensure) and actual skills.
2. Properly train staff, in terms of relevant knowledge, techniques, attitudes, and dress and shoe codes, and assign tasks only based on demonstrated abilities.
3. Monitor staff performance, both clinically and administratively, using agency policies and procedures as a guide.
4. Take corrective action, such as reassignment, suspension, or termination, where staff performance demands such action.

Communication Breakdown

Another important negligence risk in home care is the possibility of client injury caused by inadequate communication of treatment-relevant information among agency staff or between the home care agency and other providers who are involved in the care of the client.

Each home care agency must devise, implement, and monitor an effective system for communication of information necessary for client care to all staff, both within and outside the home care agency, who are involved in the care of that client (while, of course, safeguarding the client from unauthorized release of personal information). The communication system within agency staff and between the agency and independent contractors should be concerned with background information and treatment plans from the referral source, physician orders (admitting, standing, and special treatment orders), and unanticipated changes in the client condition that compel rapid action. The agency's communication system must be timely and accurate in getting information to the party(ies) (for instance, the physician or nurse) who is authorized to give or carry out orders (Jernigan, 1987). Periodic spot audits of the agency's communication system are advisable.

A home care agency may also be held legally liable for negligence in failing to communicate properly with its clients, when client harm results from that deficiency. The agency's responsibility to communicate with the client (or the client's surrogate) in the context of obtaining informed consent for various interventions has already been discussed in Chapter 3. However, the agency's ongoing communication responsibilities to the client go far beyond the relatively narrow confines of informed consent. For instance, when the home care nurse does not provide adequate, clear instructions to the client concerning the taking of medication, and the medication is taken improperly with a resulting overdose, a court may find the agency liable for negligence in its communication responsibilities (O'Neil, 1988).

The entire area of client and family teaching and training is replete with potential problems, not the least of which is ensuring that instructions are presented in an accurate, consistent manner. The following factors constrain the home care staff's attempts to educate the client and family:

- Lack of time.
- Different learning styles of client or family.
- Not ready to learn—lack of motivation.
- Past experiences of client or family.

The home care agency can reduce the effect of these constraints on the teaching–learning process by providing training information in a variety of formats. For example, information on tracheal suctioning can be developed into a workbook format, a checklist format, or a videotape. Audiovisual tapes have the added advantage of providing accurate, consistent, and cost-effective delivery of information. This also reduces the time involved in client–family instruction as they can return to the written materials or videotape as often as they need to without the actual physical presence of the nurse or therapist. Regardless of the method, all client and family training should be carefully documented along with their ability to comprehend and successfully demonstrate what they have learned. This is particularly important in the case of complex equipment. Documentation of this teaching process and the progress of the client or caregiver in learning how to use the equipment is recommended (Perdew, 1986). A safety checklist should be left in the home for the agency staff or caregiver to complete daily, to ensure that essential safety checks have been conducted and recorded (Jernigan, 1987).

An agency's communication obligations grow out of common-law tort principles predicated on the agency–client relationship and are also based on requirements in federal and state law and voluntary standards to keep the client fully informed about his or her condition and care. Home care agencies should develop and implement written policies and procedures for carrying out these responsibilities and should conduct regular in-service training sessions to ensure compliance by staff.

The foregoing discussion explores generic areas of possible negligence liability of home care agencies toward their clients. Application of some of these generic principles to particlar risk situations is explored later in this chapter and elsewhere in this book.

PRODUCTS LIABILITY

Home care today increasingly involves the use of complex and sophisticated medical equipment. Home care agencies commonly supervise the use of oxygen, suction machines, home ventilators, pacemaker communication devices, alternating pressure mattresses, apnea monitors, and electric beds, among many others. Many agencies also deal with complex machines designed to treat orthopedic problems or to provide clients with or monitor the use of invasive devices delivering hyperalimentation or chemotherapy.

A variety of problems can occur with the use of medical equipment (even assuming the equipment is appropriately prescribed in the first place) that can place the agency at legal risk if the client suffers injury. The machinery can fail to function properly as a result of a defect in the equipment itself. Conversely, the machinery may be manufactured properly but installed incorrectly. Even when correctly manufactured and installed, equipment may malfunction when a professional or paraprofessional uses it improperly, either because of lack of knowledge or skill or because of carelessness in the particular instance. Finally, and this is especially applicable to the home care setting the equipment may malfunction because the client or family caregiver who is attempting to use it does something improper, either through carelessness or because of inadequate training by the home care agency. In any of these scenarios, the consequences for the client who is dependent on the equipment may be serious and litigation may be expected. Let us examine a specific case involving equipment malfunction and highlight the home care provider's responsibilities.

Case 9–1. The Malfunctioning Ventilator

Paula is a posttraumatic-injury quadraplegic. Paula is ventilator-dependent and receives sixteen hours per day of skilled care while her husband, Ed, is at work and her teen-age daughter is in school. The manufacturer of Paula's particular model of volume ventilator has notified all durable medical equipment (DME) suppliers that this model has an unexplainable tendency to stop functioning completely for up to four minutes and then will resume functioning. Paula's DME supplier has in turn notified the home care agency on Paula's case.

The DME supplier is in the process of having all its inventory of this type of ventilator serviced, but the DME supplier does not have enough machines to remove all the ventilators at once. The home care nurses on Paula's case have been informed of the potential problem with the ventilator. Paula has a backup ventilator in the home with a backup power source. There is also an ambu bag and a separate source of oxygen to manually respirate Paula if necessary. The nurses are prepared to switch machines should the ventilator fail.

One night Paula's ventilator stops functioning. The nurse on duty quickly begins to bag Paula and calls to Ed for assistance in changing ventilators. Ed takes over respirating Paula and the nurse proceeds to switch ventilators. Perhaps because Ed is anxious about the ventilator malfunction, he bags Paula too rapidly and she proceeds to have a series of seizures. The nurse manages Paula during her seizures as well she can while Ed calls for an ambulance. Neither the nurse nor Ed are sure if or for how long Paula was without sufficient oxygen.

If Paula has sustained damages from lack of sufficient oxygen, who is responsible: the home care agency; the nurse; the DME supplier; the ventilator manufacturer; or Ed?

The ventilator manufacturer and the DME supplier appear here to have acted reasonably under the circumstances. Upon discovering the problem, the manufacturer quickly notified the DME supplier, which in turn quickly warned the home care agency so that appropriate precautions could be taken. In addition, the DME supplier worked to remedy the situation as quickly as feasible. The home care agency and its nurses took a variety of precautions in anticipation of the sort of emergency that took place. Once the emergency actually developed, the nurse on duty appears to have acted consistently with professional standards.

The problem here is with Ed's performance during the emergency. Ed will not be sued by Paula for two reasons. First, he is her husband. Second (and maybe more important in the modern era), he is not a health professional and his conduct would be held only to the standard of care of a reasonable layman, a standard he probably met. In addition, Ed carries no liability insurance for this type of activity.

However, one must ask why Ed performed poorly in this emergency. One answer may be that the home care agency and its nurses failed to prepare and train Ed properly for the type of situation that actually occurred. The home care agency and its nurses should have reasonably foreseen this scenario and worked with Ed, who they should have realized would be a vital participant, to minimize the risk of his bagging Paula too rapidly. A good argument for imposing liability on the agency and its nurses can be made for their failure to fulfill this function.

It should be remembered that the modern home care agency is considered, for legal purposes, to act as both a professional service provider and the seller of a product. The sufficiency of its professional services is judged according to a negligence standard, that is, whether those services were of a quality that would be acceptable to other reasonable, prudent home care agencies. In terms of its role as a seller (or rental agent) of a piece of equipment, the home care agency is judged according to a different (from malpractice or professional negligence) standard, namely, according to principles of *products liability*. Under products liability law, the seller of a product is legally liable for injuries caused to the purchaser if the product malfunctions as a result of inherent defects, even if there was no fault on the part of the seller. The manufacturer of the equipment and other companies in the chain of supply may also be held accountable, even without fault. Beyond liability for inherent defects, the home care agency may be held liable under a negligence standard for its errors or omissions in operating or installing the equipment or in training the client or caregiver to use it.

Therefore, it is essential for home care agencies to ensure that the complex equipment that is an integral part of home care services functions properly and is installed and operated correctly. The agency must develop, implement, and monitor policies and procedures for preventing equipment failure and providing backup support. Many home care agencies supply clients with generators, battery rechargers, and backup systems for electricity-dependent equipment, even negotiating at times with power companies regarding the delinquent bills of clients (Burda, 1986).

All equipment should be initially and then regularly inspected for proper function and condition, with these actions documented. There must be a clear, written delineation of responsibilities among equipment suppliers along the entire equipment supply chain regarding warranty, maintenance, emergency repair, backup systems, and twenty-four-hour availability. Standards have been established for the selection, inspection, monitoring, use of, and training (of both staff and clients and caregivers) of medical equipment (Joint Commission, 1988). It is more than likely that courts will adopt these industry standards as the minimum level of performance to which home care agencies will be held accountable.

Frequently, when the home care agency secures, through the manufacturer or independent supplier, equipment for the client's home use, the manufacturer or supplier will be the most knowledgeable party about that specific piece of equipment. Generally, state licensure provisions require that teaching about the use of that equipment be conducted by licensed professionals, such as a nurse or physical therapist who works for the home care agency. Licensure provisions ordinarily preclude the complete delegation of teaching responsibility from the home care agency to the manufacturer or supplier (these entities usually not being licensed as home care agencies or employing professional staff with appropriate licensure credentials). As a practical matter, however, the home care agency is well-advised to include representatives of the manufacturer or supplier in its teaching activities for the client or caregiver. Contractual arrangements between the agency and the independent contractors from whom it secures medical equipment should include stipulations obligating the manufacturer or supplier to assist home care agency staff in client and caregiver training concerning equipment provided.

RELATIONS WITH INDEPENDENT AGENCIES AND CONTRACTORS

Home care agencies traditionally have relied heavily upon independent practitioners and agencies to supply them with certain workers who provide services to clients (Kane, 1989). As noted in Chapter 6, the home care (primary) agency faces potential liability under the doctrine of *apparent or ostensible agency* when the client reasonably believed, because of the conduct of the home care agency, that the independent contractor was acting on behalf of the agency.

Apparent or Ostensible Agency

The primary agency's legal exposure under the apparent or ostensible agency doctrine may depend upon factors such as the following:

- The primary agency's role as billing agent for the independent contractor.
- The client's input or lack of input in choosing the independent contractor.
- The exclusiveness of the contract between the primary agency and the independent contractor.
- The primary agency's provision of space, equipment, and technical personnel to the contractor.
- The primary agency's legal and practical ability to control the time, manner, and method of work of the independent contractor.

Corporate Responsibility

In addition to exposure under apparent or ostensible agency principles, a home care agency also faces possible liability directly, under the principles of *corporate responsibility*, for negligence as an agency in the selection of independent contractors and the monitoring of their performance (Atkinson, 1987). The primary agency is obligated to exercise due care, according to industry standards, in its selection and monitoring of independent contractors.

Industry standards in this regard are contained in most state home care agency licensure acts. In addition, federal Medicare and Medicaid law speaks to this issue. Current federal regulations (Conditions of Participation for Home Care Agencies, Title 42 *Code of Federal Regulations*, Part 405, subpart L) require home care agency written contracts with independent suppliers of equipment or services to include at least these elements:

- Identification of acceptable professional qualifications.
- Description of the duties of indepedent contractors for client care in terms of (1) services to be performed; (2) procedures for scheduling; (3) methods for coordination, supervision, and evaluation of client care; and (4) procedures for documentation and coordination of clinical records.
- Outlining the responsibilities of the home care agency.
- Definition of admission procedures.
- Authorization of access to the contractor's records.
- Description of procedures for billing and service reimbursement.
- Making the separateness and independence of the contractor explicit.
- Specification of insurance coverage for professional liability and workers' compensation purposes.
- Implementation procedures for client confidentiality.

In addition, Congress in 1987 (Omnibus Reconciliation Act of 1987, Section 4021(1)(3)(A)) reinforced and expanded these requirements. As of this writing, the Department of Health and Human Services is working on the implementing regulations.

Further, home care standards of the JCAHO (Joint Commission, 1988) are quite specific on this topic, especially in the chapter on management and administration. JCAHO standards also require, at Standard CR.3 that, "When care or service is not provided directly by the home care organization, documentation of the contracted service is included in the home care record."

"Hold Harmless" Clauses

Another important provision that a home care agency ought to consider negotiating and including in its contracts with outside agencies is an *indemnification or "hold harmless"* clause (Burda, 1986; O'Neil, 1987) that spells out the respective rights and responsibilities of the agencies in the event of a lawsuit brought by a client. A release of liability contained in a contract between the primary agency and the independent contractor or supplier may not be effective if it purports to limit a party's responsibility for its own negligence, especially if the parties hold unequal bargaining power. However, each party may agree to be responsible only for its own acts and omissions, in return for the other party's reciprocal promise. In other words, a vendor may promise to "hold harmless" the primary agency for any injury caused by the vendor's negligence, as distinguished from the primary agency's negligence; if, in such a case, the primary agency were ordered to compensate the client for a negligently caused injury, the vendor would be obligated to indemnify or pay back to the primary agency the amount that the agency had been forced to pay the client.

An interesting model system for quality assurance of brokered services has been described from the perspective of a case manager who is responsible for contracting with home care agencies and independent vendors to achieve coordinated care programs for clients (Torres, 1988). In this model, the vendor selection process (that is, what the coordinated care program makes home care agencies and independent vendors go through in order to obtain client referrals) includes:

- Formal vendor application.
- Checking references.
- Consulting with hospital discharge planning staff, where appropriate.
- Interviewing the agency.
- Approval by corporate management.

Procedures for monitoring vendor and home care agency performance found in this model include quarterly meetings of vendors and program staff, review of incident reports involving trend analysis and sanctions if appropriate, annual evaluations, monthly client home visits and interviews, and site visits to vendor organizations (Torres, 1988). Although this model was created by and for a case manager, many of these ideas for vendor selection and monitoring are adaptable to use by home care agencies themselves in their selection and oversight of contract agencies.

Alternative Delivery Systems

A relatively new type of service arrangement involves the position of the home care agency as a vendor selling certain services through contract with an alternative delivery system (ADS) such as a health maintenance organization (HMO) or a preferred or exclusive provider organization or arrangement (PPO), (PPA), (EPO), (EPA). Such arrangements raise a variety of potential legal issues that must be anticipated and proactively addressed in the contract negotiated by the agency with the ADS.

For instance, the ADS or its designated physician, not the home care agency, generally will be authorized to make decisions prescribing home care services or supplies. Therefore, the contract should specify that the ADS will be responsible for those decisions, including decisions to terminate home care for a client, and for any negative outcomes of those decisions. The contract should also be specific regarding responsibility for liability insurance, indemnification in the case of liability, confidentiality assurances, and allocation of the duty to obtain informed consent.

In terms of the financial relationship between the home care agency and the ADS, contractual provisions should be negotiated and written concerning: risk of nonpayment, description of covered services, pricing, timing of payments, deductibles and copayments, treatment authorization requirements, utilization review, and grievance procedures, marketing, ability to subcontract, term and termination of contract, transferring clients at the end of the contract, access to books and records, renegotiation rights, and dispute resolution or arbitration.

ACCEPTANCE, TRANSFER, AND DISCHARGE OF CLIENTS

All of a home care agency's legal duties to a client grow out of the professional relationship that is formed between the two parties. Therefore, one of the most fundamental legally relevant issues that the agency confronts is whether to enter into a professional relationship with a particular individual in the first place; a related question is: At what point can an ongoing relationship with a client be terminated?

Medicare regulations require that a home care agency accept people ". . . on the basis of a reasonable expectation that the patient's medical, nursing and social needs can be met adequately by the agency in the patient's residence" (Title 42, *Code of Federal Regulations* Section 405.1223). Similarly, JCAHO home care standards provide even more detailed criteria for the admission, acceptance of referrals, the initial assessment process, and acceptance or refusal of the client (Joint Commission, 1988).

Although the home care agency may place great weight upon the recommendation of a referring physician or facility, it may not legally delegate its duty to perform an adequate assessment and to make the ultimate decision concerning admission of a new client.

New referrals must be evaluated carefully to ensure that the client is medically stable or that predictable instability, as in the case of a dying client, can be managed; that there is a desire for home care; that the home environment is suitable for the delivery of care; that the needs of the client can be safely and effectively met by the home care agency; and that satisfactory financial arrangments can be made (Haddad, 1987).

Often a predischarge hospital visit and a home assessment visit are necessary during the initial evaluation. Deficiencies—particularly regarding the lack of or adequacy of a family caregiver who will act in the absence of the home care provider—should be discussed with the physician and the client (or the client's surrogate) and carefully documented (Jernigan, 1987; Orlikoff & Vanagunas, 1988).

Information about client education and informed consent should be communicated with the client (or surrogate), both orally and in writing, at or prior to admission. Clients should be instructed on their options and other available resources and services. Realistic client, family, and physician expectations should be fostered by carefully explaining the scope and limitations of the agency's services (Gould, Ginsberg, & Perdew, 1986). In the following case study, the expectations of the family and physicians could lead to legal problems.

Case 9–2. Unrealistic Expectations of Home Care

Mary Johnson is a 5-year-old who was diagnosed with meningitis upon her admission to a local hospital's emergency room. Immediately after arriving in the emergency room, Mary had major seizure activity and a respiratory arrest. She remains on a volume ventilator for total respiratory support, has a permanent central venous line for total parenteral nutrition, and has been essentially unresponsive since her admission to the hospital 18 months ago. She is totally dependent on others for all of her care needs.

The discharge planner contacts a local home care agency that specializes in high-tech care to assess Mary's suitability for home care. Mary's insurance carrier will cover twenty-four-hour-per-day skilled nursing care in lieu of hospitalization if the cost of home care is less than acute care. Therefore, the case is financially attractive to the agency. Mary's home care needs are complex but not unusual for an agency familiar with high-tech care. What does concern the agency is the divergent views regarding Mary's prognosis.

The impetus for home care has not come from Mary's family but from Mary's physicians. There is a marked difference in how Mr. and Mrs. Johnson and Mary's physicians view her chances of recovery. Mr. and Mrs. Johnson have never given up the hope that Mary will fully recover. Mr. Johnson has built a playhouse in their backyard and states, "She'll come out of this and will be running and laughing like any other kid." The Johnsons are willing to consider home care. They tell the clinical supervisor during the initial assessment visit that they would like to have Mary at home. Mrs. Johnson states, "It would sure cut down on the trips to the hospital. However, we would want you to do everything possible to help Mary. She's gotten kind of bad several times and the doctors and nurses have been able to get her stabilized. We wouldn't accept anything less at home."

Mary's physicians, on the other hand, hold little hope for any sort of recovery to a meaningful existence. Mary appears to be in a persistent vegetative state. The physicians have attempted to present this prognosis to the Johnsons, but they refuse to listen. The physicians are frustrated in their work with the Johnsons. They feel that treatment is futile and unduly burdensome for Mary. However, they feel compelled to cooperate with the Johnsons' request for aggressive treatment because of legal concerns. The nurses and the therapists in the hospital are reluctant to care for Mary for two reasons. Most are afraid of the Johnsons' constant scrutiny and criticism of their care. One nurse commented, "With the family in there all the time, it's hard to work. They know a lot about her care and are very critical if you deviate even slightly from the routine they know."

Others feel that Mary is already "dead" and the most humane action would be to cease all life-sustaining treatment. At the very least, the majority of the hospital staff caring for Mary agree that no aggressive treatment should be instituted if, and more likely when, Mary has another crisis. The home care agency must determine if Mary and her family are suitable candidates for home care.

The legal issues in this case are considerably simpler to resolve than the ethical and psychological ones. In legal terms, first, it should be emphasized that the home care agency is under no obligation to accept Mary as a client; the decision to do so would be voluntary on their part. If the agency were to undertake Mary's care and there were a bad outcome, the possibility of a negligence suit being filed by the parents cannot be dismissed, given their apparent predisposition to be critical of Mary's care and the psychological stresses bearing upon them. However, the likelihood of such a lawsuit resulting in a finding of provider liability (or even the likelihood of a competent plaintiff's attorney taking such a case on a contingency fee basis) is much smaller. Assuming the medical prognosis is accurate, it would be extremely difficult for the parents to prove by a preponderance of evidence that any negligence (even assuming there were negligence) on the provider's part was the proximate cause of injury to Mary, who was already destined to remain at best in a persistent vegetative state.

In ethical terms, the home care agency will need to decide whether it can provide a better quality of care and quality of life for both Mary and her parents in a home care situation than she can receive in the hospital. Do the likely benefits of home care outweigh the foreseeable burdens, looked at from the perspective of Mary and her family? Will the parents' oversight and attitude engender an anxiety that would jeopardize the quality of care? Would taking Mary on as a client jeopardize the agency's ability to care properly for other clients with more potential for benefit?

The other side of the coin is determining under what circumstances a home care agency may transfer or discharge a client for whom it has been caring. Since clients may suffer adverse physical and mental reactions (sometimes called "transfer trauma") as a result of such changes in status, care in making and implementing these decisions is needed.

In accepting a client for care, a home care agency generally becomes, in effect, a case manager for that client (at least insofar as home-care-related services are concerned). In terminating a relationship with a client, the agency must be careful to avoid abandoning the client—that is, leaving the client who continues to need home care services in the lurch without adequate access to a competent source of care.

> Many providers are frightened by the notion that they cannot legally end a normal contractual relationship with the patient. They feel they are on a treadmill and will never be able to discharge the patient to any other care setting or basically to a no-care setting. The answer is, with a few exceptions dealing with licensure problems, that the caregiver does have the right to end a relationship with a patient. If the contract is not fulfilled, the caregiver does not have a perpetual, ongoing responsibility to provide services in the absence of compensation. (Randall, 1989, pp. 10–11)

Consider the following case that highlights the concern of abandonment and the differing responsibilities of the home care providers involved with the case.

Case 9–3. A Question of Abandonment

Mrs. Katz's 3-month-old daughter, Melanie, was born with several severe handicaps as a result of a lack of prenatal care and a difficult delivery complicated by Mrs. Katz's reluctance to consent to a caesarean section. Melanie is small for gestational age and has a tracheostomy and a gastrostomy for enteral feedings. Mrs. Katz has four other children under the age of 12 at home. Her mother assists in the care of the other children while Mrs. Katz is at the hospital.

Mrs. Katz is an excellent care provider for Melanie and wants to take her home. Melanie is eligible for Medicaid coverage for sixteen hours per day of skilled nursing care. Several home care agencies are contacted to assess Melanie's case. A detailed schedule is outlined for Melanie's care from 3 PM to 7 AM. Mrs. Katz chooses the Better Care Home Care agency to provide care for Melanie.

The Better Care clinical supervisor makes a home visit the day before discharge. The Katz residence is in one of the older housing projects in the community. The apartment is small but clean. The clinical supervisor notices several young men hanging about in groups around the housing project. Mrs. Katz lives on the edge of a high-crime area. Several gang-related shootings have occurred less than five blocks from the Katz apartment.

Better Care begins service delivery for Melanie and everything goes well for the first week. The second week, the 3–11 PM nurse calls the Better Care administrator on call at midnight to inform him that she will no longer care for Melanie and wants to be taken off the case. The nurse had been harrassed and "pushed around" by six adolescent males on the way to her car. She was not hurt but was terribly frightened.

After this incident, one nurse after another refuses to accept an assignment on Melanie's case. Better Care had just enough qualified nurses to accept an assignment on Melanie's case. At first, Mrs. Katz was able to care for Melanie when the agency was not able to cover the night shifts. As the weeks progress, there are fewer and fewer nurses willing to work on the case. Mrs. Katz is exhausted and states, "I'm afraid I'll do something stupid because I'm so tired." Better Care reluctantly suggests that perhaps another home care agency might be able to staff the case more consistently. Mrs. Katz agrees and asks Better Care to make some contacts with other qualified agencies in the community.

Unfortunately, when the other agencies hear about the location of the client's home, they admit that they will have an equally difficult time finding nursing staff willing to go there at night. Mrs. Katz wants to keep Melanie at home if at all possible. Finally, the Good Care Home Care agency decides that they can accept Melanie's case. However, they have had little experience with high-tech care. Can Better Care legally disharge their responsibility at this time?

A client may be discharged to an equivalent or more appropriate setting but may not be merely dropped. To avoid liability for client abandonment or dumping, the agency must develop and implement a satisfactory discharge planning program (Coleman, 1988). The JCAHO standards for home care provide specific guidelines for the transfer and discharge of clients (Joint Commission, 1988).

The process of planning the client's eventual discharge from the home are agency cannot begin too early. Ideally, discharge planning should begin immediately upon the initial assessment visit, to help identify the goals of home care and what post-home-care services will be needed and how best to obtain them (Gould, Ginsberg, & Perdew, 1986). Clients and families who have been kept involved in the discharge planning process all along the way are much less likely to feel abandoned when the relationship is terminated. Clients and families must be informed about other funding sources, community and social services, and further alternatives once they are no longer in need of or eligible for home care. It is important to document all discharge planning efforts and alternatives suggested (Jernigan, 1987).

In the case of Mrs. Katz, Better Care made a reasonable effort to transfer Melanie's care appropriately, rather than abandoning her by leaving her "high and dry" without access to an adequate source of care that she needs. Better Care has an obligation to be sure that the provider to whom Melanie is transferred is competent and appropriate. From a legal perspective, this does not impose on Better Care an obligation to set up an extensive, independent, case-by-case evaluation and accreditation system for each prospective provider–client match. Rather, Better Care satisfies its minimal legal requirements by verifying that Good Care has a state license in good standing. Any decision to look beyond state licensure in deciding upon the appropriateness of the transfer, unless Better Care has specific knowledge or notice of particular quality problems involving Good Care, would be voluntary on Better Care's part.

ABUSE AND NEGLECT BY CAREGIVERS

The incidence of child abuse is not really known, since many cases go unrecognized, but it appears to be on the increase in our society. When children are beaten, neglected, locked in closets, or turned into objects for sexual satisfaction, it is the violation of the child abuse laws and other similar statutes that make it a criminal offense and allows the abuser to be punished. It is also the same statutes that require that such crimes be reported (Calloway, 1986). Children are not the only victims of abuse and neglect.

In the late 1970s, research studies began documenting a new facet of maltreatment, maltreatment of the elderly, often at the hands of their adult children or other caregivers. "In many ways, this maltreatment is similar to others forms of domestic violence such as spouse or child abuse" (Quinn, 1985).

Home care organizations must have clear written policies and procedures regarding the detection and reporting by agency staff of suspected client abuse by caregivers or others in the home. In virtually every jurisdiction, statutes mandate the reporting of good faith, reasonable suspicion of child or adult abuse to designated state protective service authorities (O'Neil, 1988). These laws vary widely in their definitions of abuse and neglect, as well as in the standards they provide for reporting, in the penalties for failure to report, and in the types of immunity provided for those who do report (Quinn, 1985).

Failure to comply with mandatory reporting requirements may subject the home care agency and individual staff members involved to criminal misdemeanor prosecution; in a few states, failure to report abuse is classified as a felony, although prosecutions are quite rare. In addition, the agency could face possible civil litigation brought by or on behalf of an abused client, where the argument is made that a timely report to protective services authorities could have prevented or mitigated some of the later abuse. It is important to remember that mandated reporting of suspected abuse does *not* depend upon the permission of the client and must occur even over the client's objection.

The legal definitions of abuse and neglect are not that much help in delineating circumstances under which intervention by the home care provider and by the state are both justified and required (Callahan, 1988). The home care provider is in the position of being privy to all sorts of family conflicts *and* having the responsibility of sorting out which conflicts represent abuse and neglect and which are merely the normal arguments and hassles of family life. Home care personnel may identify with the stress experienced by a family in cases of abuse, which may result in a reluctance to report the incident to the appropriate authorities. A distinction, therefore, is necessary between deliberate abuse and unintentional harm to vulnerable children and elders.

> Most instances of abuse are not intentional, but result from the accumulation of stress and limited resources for providing care. In many cases, caregivers do not recognize their abusiveness; those who acknowledge it often are at a loss as to how to stop their harmful behavior. (Hooyman & Lustbader, 1985)

The home care provider may find itself increasingly involved in identifying unintentional harms to clients and working with the family to develop better coping methods and providing alternative services and support.

The home care provider's ethical obligations may go beyond what is required by law in the area of abuse. Home care providers should be able to recognize those conditions that predispose to elder abuse. "Home care workers need to better familiarize themselves with the signals [of abuse] so that they can begin to intervene at a point that maximizes support and minimizes disruption and emotional suffering" (DeRenzo, 1989, p. 12).

AIDS

The advent of the highly contagious and devastating disease acquired immune deficiency syndrome (AIDS) and the certainty that clients with this disease will be candidates for home care raise a host of legal issues concerning discrimination claims, confidentiality, negligence in care, and the rights and duties of agency staff.

Fear and prejudice among agency staff are the major problems home care providers face in coping with AIDS clients. To dispel these fears and corollary legal risks, the home care agency should proactively develop a written, specific standard operating procedure for treating infectious disease clients; JCAHO home care standards contain a detailed chapter on safety management and infection control (SI) that can be used as a model for developing such a policy along with the Centers for Disease Control universal precautions by health care workers (Joint Commission, 1988; Centers for Disease Control, 1982).

Of equal importance is the education of staff at all levels in the home care agency. Education may take the form of lectures that address the medical issues and virus transmissibility and small group sessions led by a knowledgeable individual who can clear up misinformation and facilitate discussion on a deeper level about values and fear of death. These educational sessions should be repeated at least every 3 months (or more, depending on staff turnover). The agency must also engage in close monitoring of AIDS clients, special education of family members or (especially likely with this population group) nonfamily significant others, and special steps to ensure confidentiality as much as feasible.

MEDICATION AND INTRAVENOUS THERAPY

Delivering medications and intravenous therapies in the home care setting presents special challenges in addition to the usual problems of proper administration and monitoring. For one thing, it becomes more difficult than in the hospital to monitor and detect medications or other treatments that are missed either because of accident or intentional noncompliance. In addition, complications of treatment such as infections or drug reactions may take longer to detect. Home care agencies must devise systems for addressing these problems, in terms of improved communications, training of staff and caregivers, informed consent, monitoring new procedures or drug regimens, and emergency reactions to detected problems.

RESPIRATORY THERAPIES

Particular legal risks concerning respiratory therapies (including ventilators, apnea monitors, and ancillary respiratory therapy equipment) include those associated with product and vendor selection, failure of the product when it is being used properly, and improper use of equipment, as a result either of improper training or of accident, by caregivers or home care agency staff. Risk management strategies in this area should include: testing and regular rechecking of equipment; backup equipment and power sources; periodic equipment maintenance; clear labels and instructions; proper selection and training of staff; screening and training of clients and caregivers, including a physical evaluation of the home environment. It is also important to routinely monitor equipment performance and client problems.

CONFIDENTIALITY

As a general proposition, the home care agency and its staff are obligated to treat as confidential any information that comes into their possession as a direct result of the agency–client relationship, regardless of the source of that information. For unauthorized release of confidential client information, a staff member may be held civilly liable in damages and the agency may be held vicariously or corporately liable. In addition, there may be sanctions for breach of confidentiality under state licensure acts.

Sharing Information Among Caregivers

There are numerous exceptions to the general confidentiality rule. One pertinent exception permits the sharing of relevant client information among various health care providers who are contributing to the client's care. We have already underscored the importance of timely, accurate, full communication among providers in the interests of maintaining and coordinating continuity of care; clients who "fall between the cracks" are one of the biggest clinical and legal dangers in home care.

It is advisable to obtain and document the client's (or surrogate's) written permission for information exchange among providers involved in the client's care; in the absence of this formality, however, there ordinarily is an implied permission that authorizes the sharing. Even though authorized, either explicitly or implicitly, this information sharing should be accomplished in a careful manner, being sure that only those agencies that have a legitimate need for access are provided it, and even then that only information necessary to effect proper care is transmitted.

Release of Information to Insurers

A second broad exception to the confidentiality doctrine occurs when the client or client's surrogate authorizes the release of information to a third party, such as an insurance company. Since confidentiality is a legal right that belongs personally to the client (and *not* to the provider), it is up to the client (or surrogate) to claim or waive (give up) that right. Client authorization of information release and details relating to specific instances of release to third parties should be documented clearly in the client's home care record.

Client Access to Records

In a related vein, there will be instances when a client him- or herself (or client's surrogate) will ask to see his or her own home care record. The agency should have a written policy on processing such a request. This is common in home care as the clinical record, nurses' notes and flow sheets, are often kept in the home and so clients and family members have easier access to it. There is no legal prohibition against sharing accurate information with a client. Moreover, statutes and court decisions throughout the United States establish that, although the original *physical, tangible* client records are the property of the health care provider who created the records, the client has a right to the *information* that is contained in those records. Since a client who is determined to know what information is contained in the record will eventually secure that information—through legal process if necessary—it is in the home care agency's interest to comply with the client's request in a manner that, as much as possible, bolsters rather than antagonizes the client–agency relationship.

PAIN MANAGEMENT

Many home care services are palliative in nature, aimed more at relief of pain and providing comfort for clients than cure. The issue of pain management at home is important to a variety of clients but especially the advanced cancer client.

> Estimates are that from 50–80% of advanced cancer patients will experience moderate to severe pain. The current trend toward decreased hospitalization and increased use of outpatient services has resulted in the management of the complex cancer pain syndrome at home. (Ferrell & Patterson, 1987, p. 23).

Pain management raises particular legal concerns about labeling, dispensing, and safeguarding of controlled substances under federal and state requirements, drug dependency by clients, the possibility of overdosing, the misuse by family members or friends of drugs prescribed for the client, and the possibility of drug theft from the pharmacy, delivery service, or client. The agency must develop and implement policies and procedures to ensure compliance with federal and state drug laws and to make certain that controlled substances are properly handled.

The client and family must be thoroughly trained in the administration, actions, and side effects of all pain medication. It is particularly important in the assessment visit to ascertain if there is any history of drug abuse in the family. In cases of past drug abuse by family members or significant others who live in the home, it is prudent not to administer pain medication in the home.

The home care agency staff should be adequately trained in the proper administration of pain medication in cases of chronic pain, which are the majority of cases in home care. Many health care professionals are overly concerned about drug addiction when treating clients in chronic pain. This concern has led physicians to underestimate effective dose ranges, overestimate the danger of addiction, and overestimate the drug's duration of action. The client is often left with erratic and inadequte pain management. Concerns about addiction in the client with terminal cancer are irrelevant, and those about respiratory depression (a common side effect of narcotic analgesics) should be secondary to relief of pain (Angell, 1982).

New dispensing systems for narcotic analgesics, such as implantable reservoirs (including intraspinal narcotic delivery systems), implantable continuous infusion pumps, and client controlled analgesia delivery systems all decrease the possibility of overdosing, reduce problems of accounting for single-dose vials of medication (as the dose is given or dispensed in a cartridge all at one time), and are easier to manage by clients and family members. Even with these improvements in drug administration, the home care agency needs to establish a procedure that will provide proof of delivery and use of all narcotics. Finally, it is important to keep flowing the lines of communication between the home care agency and prescribing physician.

DEFENSES TO NEGLIGENCE CLAIMS

Several different kinds of legal defenses are available to counter a claim of negligence that might be brought against a home care agency. One type of defense is *procedural*, such as the expiration of the applicable statute of limitations. Another category of defense would be *denial* of one or more of the plaintiff's essential elements of proof:

- The duty or standard of care.
- Deviation from that duty (fault).
- Injury or damage, or causation.

In home care settings, it may be especially difficult for clients to establish the element of *causation* where the defendant may be able to argue that fault by the client or caregiver was just as likely as improper conduct by the home care agency to have brought the client's injury (Johnson, 1988).

Assumption of Risk

A home care agency might also argue the defense of assumption of risk in opposition to a negligence claim. Under the assumption of risk principle, a defendant is relieved of responsibility where the plaintiff voluntarily assumed a known risk that materialized and caused injury. Thus, if a client is told that he or she may suffer a negative reaction to a specific drug and such a reaction does occur, the client cannot blame on the home care agency the materialization of the risk that the client voluntarily and knowingly assumed.

Contributory or Comparative Negligence

Under the contributory negligence defense, a defendant is not legally liable, despite negligence, if the plaintiff was also at fault and the injury was caused at least in part by the plaintiff's error. Hence, if the home care agency improperly installs a piece of equipment in the home, but the caregiver makes the situation worse by using the equipment in an improper manner, in a contributory negligence jurisdiction the home care agency would be relieved of responsibility. Many states in the last several years have moved to a comparative negligence standard, in which the complete defense afforded by the contributory negligence rule is replaced by a rule that relieves negligent defendants of responsibility only to the extent that the plaintiff's own fault contributed to his or her injury.

In the health care field generally, courts tend to disfavor the assumption of risk and contributory or comparative negligence defenses, exhibiting a bias toward assigning responsibility to the health care provider. The extent to which the courts may apply these defenses in the home health arena has yet to be established through definitive test cases.

DOCUMENTATION

Throughout this and other chapters, we have emphasized the importance of complete, timely, accurate documentation of client care. Adequate client records are essential not only for liability prevention and claims defense, but also for licensure, certification, and reimbursement purposes, especially related to quality assurance, coordination of services, and continuity of care. Federal and state law set minimum requirements for record keeping and JCAHO standards contain an entire chapter (Chapter 4, Home Care Record) on the subject. When it comes to client care documentation, one is best guided by the lawyer's adage, "If it's not written, you didn't do it!" (Sutton, 1988).

Special documentation challenges arise in home care because the supervision of care often is at a distance, two or more providers may share responsibility for client care, physician orders regularly are obtained by telephone, environmental factors and interventions by family members must be taken into account, and many of the personnel are either independent contractors or employed part-time. Specific areas where special documentation efforts must be exerted by the home care agency include:

- Admission assessments.
- Informed consent.
- Verbal orders.
- Emergency responses, including notifying physician of instability.
- Charting of ongoing stable conditions as well as any unusual developments (because the client who does well today may suddenly do poorly tomorrow, and the home care agency may be blamed).

RISK MANAGEMENT STRATEGIES

Many different kinds of legal risks are alluded to in this book, as well as strategies for addressing those risks. There are basically four things that can be done by any organization that is confronted by legal risks: (1) avoidance; (2) reduction of probability of occurrence or severity of loss; (3) transfer, through insurance and "hold harmless" agreements; and (4) retention, by choice or necessity.

Many home care agencies historically have engaged in some risk management activities, mainly through their financial offices, such as safety programs, insurance coverage, asset management, and corporate structuring to reduce legal exposure (Gould, Ginsberg, & Perdew, 1986). Today, however, the home care industry has become too large, complex, and sophisticated—and the legal climate has become too precarious—to continue risk management on a piecemeal, *ad hoc* basis. Home care agencies must think seriously about implementing comprehensive, formal risk management systems designed to reduce legal (and thus financial) exposure resulting from injuries to clients. Ideally, such systems should be closely integrated with the agency's quality assurance program (Perdew, 1986).

A complete dissertation on the structure and mechanics of a risk management system is beyond the scope of this book (see generally Kapp, 1987a; Orlikoff & Vanagunas, 1988). At the least, liability insurance coverage or a funded self-insurance program, as well as extensive staff education, should be included.

Incident Reports

In addition, an occurrence or incident reporting and follow-up system is an essential building block of risk management. Incident reports are written, contemporaneous records of events that function to: (1) inform management so that it can identify trends and take preventive or corrective action; and (2) inform legal counsel so that he or she can evaluate particular risks and prepare to prevent or defend a lawsuit (Connaway, 1986). There are several strategies for protecting confidentiality of incident reports under the attorney–client privilege and the attorney–work product doctrine.

Another component of a risk management system that is especially important in home care, where supervision is so diffuse and care and supplies are often provided for on a contractual basis, is a system to ensure the opportunity for clients and caregivers to provide *feedback* directly to management about their perceptions of the quality of services received (Applebaum & Christianson, 1988). These perceptions—particularly dissatisfactions—should then be investigated and acted upon by agency management to head off or mitigate potential problems and to maintain good relations generally with clients and their families. In the final analysis, maintaining good relations with those to whom the agency owes a duty—and thus those who might qualify as potential plaintiffs in a malpractice lawsuit—represents the most effective risk management strategy of all.

REFERENCES

American Hospital Association, Hospital Research and Education Trust, Institute on Quality of Care and Patterns of Practice. (1987). *Managing Risks*

and Quality in Hospital-Sponsored Home Care. Chicago: American Hospital Association.
Angell, M. (1982). The quality of mercy. *New England Journal of Medicine, 106*: 98–99.
Applebaum, R., & Christianson, J. (1988). Using case management to monitor community-based long term care. *Quality Review Bulletin, 14*(7): 227–231.
Atkinson, S.C. (1987). Note, Medicare 'cost containment' and home health care: Potential liability for physicians and hospitals. *Georgia Law Review, 21*: 901–927.
Burda, D. (1986). Five future areas of liability risks haunt providers. *Hospitals, 60*(22): 48–53.
Callahan, J.J. (1988). Elder abuse: Some questions for policymakers. *The Gerontologist, 28*: 453–458.
Calloway, S.D. (1986). *Nursing Ethics and the Law.* Eau Claire, Wis: Professional Education Systems, Inc.
Centers for Disease Control. (1982). Acquired immune deficiency syndrome (AIDS): Precautions for clinical and laboratory staffs. *Morbidity and Mortality Weekly Report, 31*(November 5): 577–80.
Code of Federal Regulations Title 42. (August 1989). Medicare Program; *Home Health Agencies: Conditions of Participation*; Department of Health and Human Services.
Coleman, S. (1988). Discharge planning for the home health agency. In P.A. O'Hare & M.A. Terry (Eds.), *Discharge Planning: Strategies for Assuring Continuity of Care.* Rockville, Md: Aspen Publishers.
Connaway, N.I. (1986). Incident reports in home health agencies. *Home Healthcare Nurse, 4*(3): 9–10.
Darling v Charleston Community Memorial Hospital, 33 I11 2d 326, 211 NE 2d 253 (1965), *cert. denied*, 383 US 946 (1966).
DeRenzo, E.G. (1989). Elder abuse: Ethical theory in every day practice. *Caring, 8*(3): 10–12.
Ferrell, B.R., & Patterson, B. (1987). Pain at home: Implications for home care providers. *Caring, 6*(11): 22–25.
Gould, E.J., Ginsberg, A., & Perdew, S.R. (1986). Home care challenge. *Caring, 5*(9): 74–83.
Greenberg, R.B. (1986). Legal implications of home health care by nonprofit hospitals. *American Journal of Hospital Pharmacy, 43*: 386–391.
Haddad, A. (1987). *High Tech Home Care: A Practical Guide.* Rockville, Md: Aspen Publishers.
Hooyman, N.R., & Lustbader, W. (1985). *Taking Care.* New York: The Free Press.
Jernigan, D.K. (1987). Managing risk in the home care setting. *Home Care Economics, 1*(2): 46–52.
Johnson, S.H. (1988). Who sets the standards for home healthcare? *Health Progress, 69*(11): 20–21.
Joint Commission on Accreditation of Healthcare Organizations. (1988). *Standards for the Accreditation of Home Care.* Chicago: Joint Commission on Accreditation of Healthcare Organizations.
Kane, N.M. (1989). The home care crisis of the nineties. *The Gerontologist, 29*(1): 24–31.

Kapp, M.B. (1987). Legal issues. In A.M. Haddad, *High Tech Home Care: A Practical Guide*. Rockville, Md: Aspen Publishers.

Kapp, M.B. (1987a). *Preventing Malpractice in Long Term Care: Strategies for Risk Management*. New York: Springer Publishing Company.

Omnibus Reconciliation Act of 1987, Public Law 100-203, printed at *Congressional Record, 133*(205) Part III, December 24, 1987.

O'Neil, E.A. (1987). Legal issues. In D. Lerman (Ed.), *Home Care: Positioning the Hospital for the Future*. Chicago: American Hospital Publishing, Inc.

O'Neil, E.A. (1988). Legal aspects of home health management. In L.E. Benefield (Ed.), *Home Health Management*. Englewood Cliffs, NJ: Prentice-Hall, Inc.

Orlikoff, J.E., & Vanagunas, A.M. (1988). *Malpractice Prevention and Liability Control for Hospitals*. Chicago: American Hospital Publishing, Inc.

Perdew, S.R. (1986). Litigation in home care: What the future holds. *Caring*, *5*(9): 84–88.

Quinn, M.J. (1985). Elder abuse and neglect raise new dilemmas. *Generations*, *10*(2): 22–25.

Randall, D.A. (1989). Patients' rights and provider accountability. *PRIDE Institute Journal of Long Term Home Health Care*, *8*(2): 4–11.

Roach v Kelly Health Care, 742 P 2d 1190 (Or App 1987).

Sutton, S. (1988). *Home Health Nursing Manual: Procedures and Documentation*. Baltimore: The Williams & Wilkins Co.

Torres, M.S. (1988). Quality assurance of brokered services. *Quality Review Bulletin*, *14*(6): 187–192.

Chapter 10

Organizational Values

Amy Marie Haddad

One of the fundamental goals of home care is to deliver the best possible care to each client and family. However, it is often difficult to determine what is the "best" possible care or course of action. In order to determine what is best, one must make value judgments. Values clarification is necessary for understanding the extent to which a person's beliefs and attitudes influence decisions made in health care, whether these decisions are made by clients, family members, nurses, aides, or home care administrators (Thompson & Thompson, 1985).

Just as individuals need to know themselves—their beliefs and values—so do organizations. Home care organizations, regardless of profit or nonprofit status, have a set of values and expect their employees to know, internalize, and act on these values. This chapter will explore the values inherent in home care and propose methods for developing and nurturing an organizational ethos. Finally, practical suggestions will be offered to assist the home care provider in the establishment of an institutional ethics committee.

VALUES INHERENT IN HOME CARE

Ethics is concerned with rights, responsiblities, needs, and values. In the day-to-day business of home care, ethical considerations and values may seem like vague abstractions compared to the all too real need to balance the budget. It appears to many that a values-oriented approach has been replaced by a bottom-line approach in home care. It is sometimes difficult to get managers to take values systems seriously. Yet, Peters and Waterman (1982) found in their study of "excellent" companies, that there was consistent attention to values and a clarity of purpose and that the process of value shaping was taken seriously. With this in mind, let us proceed to an examination of the meaning of home care and its values and practical implications.

Meaning of Home Care

Home care is a unique, hands-on kind of care. Home care summons up visions of familiar surroundings, warmth, and security. Family members poignantly describe the intimacy of home care: "And as my mother lost her appetite, lost her ability to read, lost her will to fight, Marilyn [a home care nurse] also baked zucchini bread for her, read to her, arrived in the morning with flowers from her garden" (Jaret, 1984, p. 61). Home care providers are encouraged to provide personal, individualized care.

> We should be able to call by name the little grey kitty keeping watch on her master's death bed; to be aware that young Stephen recently celebrated his bar mitzvah; and to know that our patient's granddaughter was accepted in the cheerleading squad. (Ufema, 1984, p. 5)

These portrayals of home care reveal much more than just the events depicted. The word *home* in itself is extremely potent, conjuring up deeply personal and subconscious meanings. Contrast these meanings of home care with an institutional setting. One is hospitalized, but one *receives* home care. The semantics of these statements is not accidental. In the acute care setting, patients are passive recipients. Treatments and procedures are performed on the patient. The schedule is designed to meet the needs of the bureaucracy, not the client. As the use of sophisticated technology increases, so does the dehumanization. "A stay in the hospital exposes an individual to a condition of passivity and impotence unparalleled in adult life, this side of prison" (Gaylin, 1973, p. 22).

The following excerpt concerns a 78-year-old male client who has been admitted to an intensive care unit after a massive cerebral hemorrhage. This passage clearly distinguishes the world of the intensive care unit from the familiarity of home through the eyes of the client's grandson.

> Ten minutes later a grandchild, a thin boy in his late teens, walked stiffly into the room. He stared straight ahead as if prepared to fight the enemy which held his grandfather. The boy reached out to touch the older man's face and caught himself. He would not make this real. This was his grandfather, a man he had loved all his life. He would not give him up to the world of these ugly tubes and sterile smells. His grandpa was the smell of pipe tobacco and apples. He was the tall, balding man always telling stories. Gramps was the wisest man he'd ever known; he would not let him go. (Heron, 1987, p. 4)

Home care, unlike institutional care, is an extension of our normal lives. We have all experienced home care—a parent caring for a sick child; a neighbor bearing a pot of steaming chicken soup. These experiences with home care, no matter how unsophisticated, shape our understanding and values of what home care should be.

The home care industry has drawn heavily on these personal images of home and personal care. Home care has been marketed as the humane alternative to institutional care. Also, there are demonstrable social, psychological, and physical benefits from home care. By fostering these images and emphasizing these benefits, home care providers are thereby obligated to fulfill the expectations they create.

The Value of Clients and Families

Values are preferred stances of thinking, feeling and doing. They affect the people toward whom practice is directed, as well as the quality of home care (Lowy, 1979). Values have a significant impact on practice. True values are acted upon; they are evident in behavior. The purpose of home care is to deliver health care services to individuals and families in the home setting. The client and the family are the focus of the work. Home care providers are called to assist clients and families to integrate, restore, or improve human function. While home care providers are called to assist, they are also called to respect an individual's self-determination and decision making abilities.

> By virtue of this function or power [self-determination], people are of inestimable worth, and anyone who seeks to help another regain health must do so with reverence for this worth. The reverence and respect for the person and for the creative function are the basis for requiring informed consent and other ethical norms, such as confidentiality and truth telling, that have been stressed in the practice of medicine in recent years. (O'Rourke & Brodeur, 1989, p. 61).

This emphasis on respect for the individual informs every interaction in home care and is most obvious in the plan of care. Care is tailored to the individual needs and desires of the client and family. The home care provider must become familiar with a client's routines, likes and dislikes, and design a plan of care that suits the client. The client is not expected to dramatically adjust his or her life to the needs and the wishes of the home care provider. Though individualized care is held as an ideal in other health care settings, it is the hallmark of home care.

The task of individualizing care and respecting the independence of clients and families is not easy. In fact, it is one of the most common ethical problems in home care according to one study, which consisted of surveys, round table discussions, and telephone interviews of home care providers. The study found that at home, clients feel more secure and are much more likely to resist following orders or taking advice. "So when healthcare professionals persist and override a patient's objections, the patient is likely to perceive the act as a heavy-handed assault on his or her self-determination" (Young, Pignatello, & Taylor, 1988, p. 60).

This underlying tension between the home care provider and the client and family regarding authority and control has been discussed at length elsewhere (see Chapter 3). What is important to the present discussion is that true values are evident in behavior. If the home care provider, on an individual or organizational basis, only pays lip service to the idea of importance of respect for persons and its corollaries, conflicts over who is in charge will be common.

The Value of Service

The most obvious way of demonstrating respect for clients and families is to do a good job of caring for them. The value of a job well done is difficult to measure and is certainly the focus of great concern in the home care industry. "Controlling quality in a service business is a particularly difficult problem. Unlike manufacturing, in which one can sample what comes off the line and reject bad lots, what gets produced in service businesses and what gets consumed happens at the same time and in the same place" (Peters & Waterman, 1982, p. *xix*). The home care provider must ensure that all of its personnel are roughly adhering to the same values.

Even though models for quantitative and qualitative evaluation of service delivery are in their infancy, there is a clear, underlying service orientation in home care. This service value implies a desire and ability to help a person with impaired function so that the person can become a better human being (O'Rourke & Brodeur, 1989). The relationship between the home care provider and client must be based on trust rather than money. That is not to say that the home care provider should forget about money and exist on good will alone. The home care agency must maintain fiscal stability in order to maintain trust relationships with clients and families. Though the ability to pay enters into the relationship between the client and home care provider, it must be considered as secondary. The worth of home care is almost impossible to measure. The rewards are intangible and deeply personal. The satisfaction of helping individuals who are vulnerable and in need, on their terms and territory, is the source of values in home care.

DEVELOPING AN ORGANIZATIONAL ETHOS

The values associated with individual members of the home care team apply as well to the home care organization as a whole, be it a singly owned, nonprofit agency or a corporate chain. "Corporations are recognized by law as entities (moral persons) pursuing the same goals as individuals, although ostensibly in a more effective manner"

(O'Rourke & Brodeur, 1989, p. 65). Home care organizations must have the same primary purpose as their employees.

Webster defines *ethos*, a Greek root word for ethics, as "the distinguishing character, sentiment, moral nature, or guiding beliefs of a person, group, or institution." Tangible evidence of an organization's ethos may be hard to find. Those organizations that take their values seriously, however, know that *every* member of their organization should be able to articulate what's important, what they're about, and why they're there. This is the ethos, the moral fabric, of an organization.

Communicating Within

It is important to clearly and explicitly communicate values within an organization. One method of communication is a formal code of ethics. When an individual home care agency or a corporate chain establishes a code of ethics, they are establishing a guide for minimal performance of the agency, as a corporate person, and its individual representatives. A code of ethics is distinct from a bill of rights statement. The most widely disseminated document of this latter type is the American Hospital Association's *A Patient's Bill of Rights* (1972). The Bill affirms that a hospitalized patient has the right to:

- Considerate and respectful care.
- Reasonable continuity of care.
- Privacy.
- Protection of confidentiality.
- Reasonable response to requests.
- An explanation of charges.

When the Bill affirms that a client has the right to give informed consent or to refuse treatment, it is merely reiterating that hospitals and their representatives are subject to the same laws concerning assault and battery and negligence as any other institution or member of society (Gaylin, 1973). A home care provider, or any other health care provider, does not have the authority to grant rights to clients and families. Rights are vested in the client and family. What the home care provider does have control over is whether or not the rights of the client and family will be respected. A right is of little value if it is not respected. By focusing solely on patient's rights, the authors of the *Patient's Bill of Rights* encourage paternalism. The responsibilities of the health care provider are not clear or mandated.

A code of ethics, on the other hand, expresses basic moral principles. It reminds caregivers and managers alike that the lives and well-being of people depend on professional skills and integrity. A code of ethics provides a minimally decent standard of conduct for those in the health care professions. An example of a model code of ethics which was written for a fictious home care agency, Anytown Home Care, is presented [below]. This code has been adapted from the National Association for Home Care (NAHC) *Code of Ethics*. The significant difference between the NAHC *Code of Ethics* and the following code is that the Anytown Home Care code emphasizes the responsibilities of the home care provider rather than client rights.

Exhibit 10–1. Code of Ethics

This Code of Ethics serves to inform employees and the public as to what are acceptable guidelines for ethical conduct in the delivery of service. This Code of Ethics serves as a reminder regarding the ideals embraced by Anytown Home Care and of the duties assumed in the role of home care provider.

1. Anytown Home Care (AHC) has the responsibility to fully inform clients of all their rights and responsibilities.
2. AHC has the responsibility to provide appropriate and professional care relating to physician orders.
3. The client has the right of choice of care providers.
4. AHC has the responsibility to provide information to the client necessary to give informed consent prior to the start of any procedure or treatment.
5. The competent client has the right to refuse treatment and to be informed of the consequences of his or her decision.
6. The client's legally valid surrogates have the right to refuse treatment within the confines of the law and to be informed of the consequences of their decision.
7. AHC has the responsibility to respect the decisions of competent clients or their legally valid surrogates.
8. AHC has the responsibility to protect the privacy of each client and family.
9. AHC has the responsibility to respect the dignity of each client.
10. AHC has the responsibility to provide a timely response to a client's request for service.
11. AHC will only admit a client for service if AHC can provide safe professional care at the level of intensity needed. The client has the right to reasonable continuity of care.
12. AHC has the responsibility to inform clients within a reasonable time of anticipated termination of service or of plans for transfer of the client to another provider.

13. The client has the right to voice grievances and suggest changes in service or staff without fear of reprisal or discrimination.
14. AHC has the responsibility to fully inform clients of agency policies and charges for services, including eligibility for third-party reimbursements.
15. AHC has the responsibility to make a reasonable attempt to assist those clients whom the agency has been unable to serve in finding alernative community resources and support.

In the absence of a formal code of ethics, individual members of the home care team may turn to their particular profession's code of ethics for guidance. For example, the *Standards of Home Health Nursing Practice* state:

> The Council of Community Health Nurses accepts the ethical standards explicit in the *Code for Nurses with Interpretive Statements*. Nurses who work with home care clients encounter situations in which human rights and freedom are in jeopardy. Therefore, it is important for the rights of clients as well as nurses to be acknowledged. (American Nurses' Association, 1986, p. 3)

Generally, these specific codes do not conflict with the broader code a home care provider could develop for itself.

Key personnel, representing all levels and areas, should be involved in the drafting of a code of ethics or personalizing an existing code. The language can always be refined but the ownership that results from articulating values and what the home care provider stands for are invaluable.

It is not enough to write a code of ethics and hang it on a bulletin board. Codes are important but they need the backup of frank discussions, such as staff meetings, that alert individual employees to the ethical nature of their obligations to clients and their families. Employees and clients must feel that they can speak freely about breaches of ethical responsibility without fear of reprisal.

Not only is it important to communicate values within an organization, it is equally important to brief prospective clients and their families regarding the home care provider's values or code of ethics. This is an excellent opportunity to see if the organization's values match the client's. It is probable that in the not too distant future, health care providers, organizations, and individuals alike will have to share their moral framework for care delivery before they enter into a formal contractual relationship with the client.

Responding to External Pressure

The home care industry is an extremely competitive one. At times, it might seem that ethics are luxuries that a home care provider cannot afford if it is to survive. If a home care provider holds to the standard cited in the previous model code of ethics: "AHC will only admit a client for service if AHC can provide safe professional care at the level of intensity needed," it is possible that at times, it will not be able to accept a client. This will not stop Home Care Agency X, down the street, from accepting the same client, even though X is less qualified than the first provider. Though AHC is fulfilling its obligations, it may appear in the short run that it is losing income. However, good ethics can mean good business, as well.

High ethical standards can translate into high profits. The ethical edge in a business such as home care can enable an agency to attract talent, win loyal customers and suppliers, and earn the public's good will. This sometimes calls for letting an opportunity slip by or incurring a short-term financial loss (Berney, 1987).

Even if a home care provider stands to lose financially in a given situation, it is still important to do the right thing ethically for broader, more far-reaching reasons. Essentially, by behaving in an ethical manner the home care provider can maintain its integrity—to be true to its fundamental ideals and values—which is of direct benefit to the home care provider and its relationships with others, including employees and clients.

ESTABLISHING AN ETHICS COMMITTEE

Another means to address pressures of business and corresponding ethical matters is an ethics committee. Though the majority of ethics committees have originated in institutions, particularly hospitals, the shift of advanced technology and complex clients to home care justifies the development of ethics committees outside hospital walls. Home care ethics committees are relatively new. Whether the committee is made up of a variety of representatives from home care providers throughout a community or a single home care provider, an ethics committee can be an excellent resource in reviewing potential areas of ethical conflict and ethical decision making (Baginski, 1989).

Depending on the type and volume of cases a home care provider takes and the complexity of ethical issues, it may be in the home care provider's interest to establish its own ethics committee. If this is not feasible, the functions of an ethics committee should be delegated to an already-existing group within the organization such as a quality assurance commitee, advisory board, or board committee. Whatever form an ethics committee takes, it is important to formally charge an identified group within the organization to respond thoughtfully and systematically to ethical problems.

Why Ethics Committees?

The concept of an ethics committee is not new. There have long been ethics committees of one type or another. They have been used in hospitals where there are value conflicts that have been explicitly identified and that cannot be ignored (Annas, 1984). In the past, committees of this type have taken the following forms: (1) medical–moral committees that existed in the 1950s and 1960s to review the appropriateness of abortions and sterilization procedures; (2) patient selection committees for dialysis treatment (which were later abandoned when the federal government chose to fund all treatment for end-stage renal disease in 1972); and (3) Institutional Review Boards, which are designed to review research proposals and informed consent of subjects.

> One of the earliest uses of the term "ethics committee" appeared in the New Jersey Supreme Court's ruling in the Karen Ann Quinlan case in 1976. The court ordered the establishment of ethics committees in hospitals to review and confirm the prognosis of patients like Quinlan, judged to be in a persistent vegetative state with no reasonable hope of recovery to sapient existence. Although the court termed these committees, "ethics committees," it was actually describing "prognosis committees". (Macklin & Kupfer, 1988, p. 3; *In re Quinlan*. (1976)

Prognosis committees are not the same as ethics committees, as medical prognosis can only be determined by qualified physicians.

In 1983, the Committee on Bioethics of the American Academy of Pediatrics recommended the establishment of local ethics committees as a mechanism for assisting in decisions about critically ill newborns (American Academy of Pediatrics, 1983). The American Medical Association House of Delegates adopted guidelines for ethics committees in health care institutions in 1984 (American Medical Association Council Report, 1985).

Today, multidisciplinary ethics committees exist in the majority of hospitals. Hospital-based committees have been largely concerned with ethical issues generated by high-tech care. The focus of the committee changes as one moves to extended care and out into the community. Regardless of the setting, the general purpose of an ethics committee is to provide a structural format for individuals within an organization to increase their awareness of ethics and their application to clinical practice.

Organizing the Committee

The composition of the ethics committee will depend on the philosophy and values of the organization. It will also depend on the origin of the committee. If the committee is established by the board of directors of a home care agency, it may have a different composition from a committee established by the nursing staff. Generally, committees are multidisciplinary with representatives from nursing, medicine, law, ethics, social work, religion, and the community.

A typical committee should consist of a nurse manager, a staff nurse, a homemaker–home health aide, a physician, a therapist (physical, occupational, or speech), a social worker, a member of the clergy, an attorney, an ethicist, and one or more representatives from the community. Ordinarily, the home care agency's legal counsel should not serve on the committee because of his or her concern to limit the home care agency's liability, which may conflict with the best interest of the client and family whose case is being discussed (Drane & Roth, 1985).

An ethics consultant should be appointed to the committee. The consultant should be selected based on his or her expertise in ethics and familiarity with home care or, at a minimum, health care. The home care provider could seek out such an individual from a local university or college in the philosophy department or health sciences schools. The consultant can provide in-service education to the committee members regarding basic moral principles and ethical theories.

The total number of committee members should be kept to a dozen or less to allow for manageable group discussion. The majority of ethics committee members are volunteers who are willing to participate because of interest or expertise. The multidisciplinary model provides a broad representation of perspectives on a given issue. Ethics committees are an example of a "community of concern"—that group of persons necessary to grasp all of the essential dimensions of a given issue (Glaser, 1989).

All committee members should have training in applied ethics. An orientation session, or a series of sessions, can be used to acquaint members with terminology. Many committees spend the first year of their existence involved solely in self-education. The majority of ethics committees meet on an average of seven times per year (McCarrick & Adams, 1987).

"Some ethics committees have found that by staggering the terms of members and by employing a 'buddy system' to link the new members with the old, the openness and trust between members can be extended" (Bayley, 1986, p. 6).

Basic Functions of An Ethics Committee

A home care ethics committee can fulfill one or more of the following functions:

- Educate staff about the ethical dimensions of home care.
- Develop policies or guidelines.
- Serve as a forum for discussing conflicts regarding care decisions.
- Serve as a source of support as these difficult decisions are made.
- Review cases and offer advice to those directly involved in the case (Levine, 1984).

The mere presence of an ethics committee serves to encourage positive conscious efforts to resolve ethical problems and to prevent them from occurring in the future.

An additional function has been suggested, which ethics committees cannot avoid—standing up for moral concerns. The concern for and protection of the autonomy and dignity of individual clients and their families are two of the most important potential functions of ethics committees (Annas, 1984).

Process for Developing Policies and Guidelines

Ethics committees are in a prime position to help the home care agency establish policies where no such policies existed or where the exisiting policies are ambiguous or inadequate to meet novel situations. The impetus for policies can be internal and reflect the specific concerns of a home care agency or external, such as a federal regulation or accreditation standard. The following procedure is proposed for the thoughtful, systematic development of policies:

1. Educate committee members regarding technical and ethical issues.
2. Develop a policy based on reflection of technical and ethical issues.
3. Test the policy.
4. Finalize and approve the policy.
5. Orient personnel to the policy.
6. Review the policy periodically.

To clarify the steps in the process, the steps will be applied to the development of a policy for the decision to withhold life-sustaining treatment, specifically, do-not-resuscitate orders. The impetus for this policy is the Joint Commission on Accreditation of Healthcare Organization (JCAHO) Home Health standard HH.10, which states:

> The home organization has written policies and procedures regarding the resuscitation of patients and for documentation in the home care record, including, as appropriate, provisions for appropriate orders by the patient's/client's physician (Joint Commission, 1988).

Educate Committee Members. Committee members must be educated regarding the technical and ethical issues involved, in this case, with cardiopulmonary resuscitation (CPR). The technical information regarding do-not-resuscitate (DNR) orders should include the following information: a definition and explanation of CPR; instances in which CPR is indicated and not indicated; and the efficacy of CPR in the context of home care.

Case 10–2 provides an example of the sort of background information the committee needs to formulate a policy. Initially, the committee may have difficulty identifying the ethical issues that pertain to the policy. It is the responsibility of the ethics consultant to assist the committee in this regard, isolating the ethical concerns from other issues involved in the policy. In addition, committee members could be given pertinent literature on DNR to supplement the background information.

Exhibit 10–2. Background Information for Formalizing the Decision to Withhold Cardiopulmonary Resuscitation

Instituting cardiopulmonary resuscitation or CPR is of central concern for every health care setting. Resuscitation of a client who has suddenly stopped breathing can involve a variety of procedures. Basically, cardiopulmonary resuscitation involves artificially "breathing" for a client who has stopped breathing and circulating blood volume by manual cardiac compression in the event of cardiac cessation. If resuscitation is performed in a timely manner (within three minutes) on an otherwise strong client, a pulse and respirations can be restored and the client may eventually recover completely. In other cases, clients with a terminal diagnosis may respond to resuscitative measures but remain in a comatose state or regain consciousness to suffer through the remainder of a lingering painful illness.

Since CPR is an emergency procedure, it is essential for the client (if he or she is competent), the physician, and the entire health care team to decide in advance whether resuscitation should be initiated. This is particularly important in home care as front-line support to the resuscitative effort is not within the home and usually some distance away. In most cases, a code should be called. However, in cases in which the dying trajectory of a patient is evident and resuscitation in the event of a cardiac or pulmonary arrest would not change the trajectory to any advantage, the question of resuscitation should be seriously examined. It has even been suggested that resuscitation in some circumstances may represent a positive violation of a person's right to die with dignity.

The practice of waiting until an emergency situation to decide resuscitation status is procedurally and ethically undesirable in the acute care setting and can be disastrous in the home care setting. Open discussions with the client, family, clergy, and the home care team offers the opportunity to clarify treatment goals, acknowledge the gravity of the prognosis, and realistically deal with the dying process. If advance planning has not occurred or there is disagreement regarding the do-not-resuscitate order, the home care provider ordinarily is ethically obligated to proceed with resuscitative measures.

Develop the Policy. The committee can now move to the reflection phase of the process. The committee can either work together to draft a policy or respond to a draft policy that has been prepared by the ethics consultant. In the interest of saving time, it is often easier to respond to a draft. The policy should reflect sound clinical rationale and ethical justification for each proposed action. Exhibit 10–3 is a sample policy for formalizing the decision to withhold CPR in the case of competent adult clients.

Exhibit 10–3. Formalizing the Decision to Forego Cardiopulmonary Resuscitation In the Case of Competent Adult Clients

Shared decision making by physicians and informed, competent clients is recommended in decisions about withholding life-sustaining treatment. In this case, the life-sustaining treatment in question is cardiopulmonary resuscitation (CPR). This decision is often referred to as a "do-not-resuscitate" order or DNR order. Discussions about resuscitation status should be held in a timely manner with respect for the individual needs of the client and the family. However, the discussion should begin prior to formalizing the service agreement between the client and home care provider.

1. The health care professional must define the anticipated benefits and burdens of resuscitation and inform the client.
2. Competent, informed clients may refuse resuscitation even though others may regard this decision as unwise. Deciding whether a

treatment, such as resuscitation, is futile may be very difficult. There may be controversy over the goals of treatment. Decisions about the effectiveness of any treatment rest on imperfect information. Therefore, open, honest communication between the health care provider and client is essential to informed decision making.

3. If the client and the physician are in agreement regarding the DNR order, the physician should express this clearly, in writing, on the client's medical record for the benefit of nursing and other personnel who may be called upon to initiate or participate in CPR.
4. A written DNR order should be reassessed at least on a weekly basis and changed if necessary but only with the client's input.
5. If there is disagreement between the client and the physician, the client has the right to seek a second opinion. It would be ethically prudent for the physician in a case such as this to offer to refer the client to another physician.

   The physician and other members of the home care team should check whether changing temporary conditions might cause the client to change his or her mind (ie, pain relief, extreme depression).
6. The physician should discuss with the client whether to inform the family about the DNR decision. Ideally, the client and the family should be involved in the decision-making process jointly from the outset.

A similar policy would also need to be drafted to address DNR orders in the case of the incompetent client.

Test the Policy. The draft policy should then be routed through the communication channels of the home care agency. It is crucial that the staff most directly affected by the policy be involved in refining it. Field staff bring critical observations to policy development, as they are most directly involved in the day-to-day observations of clients and their families. Through this process of field testing, the gaps in the policy become apparent before it is officially adopted. The policy should then return to the ethics committee for revisions and final approval.

Orientation to the Policy. It is not sufficient for a policy to be written and then placed in a manual. Key staff should be given a formal orientation to the policy and its application to practice. The ethics committee should work closely with risk-management personnel quality-assurance committees whenever a policy is implemented.

Review Policy Periodically. Most ethics committees fail to review policies that have been developed. It is time-consuming and difficult to reexamine a policy that has taken considerable time to develop and approve. Nevertheless, the committee should routinely review policies in light of changes in clinical practice, standards of care, or client acuity. "The process of obtaining feedback from the staff should continue even after the policy is put into effect so that any misunderstanding on the part of the staff members acting on the policy can be resolved" (Ross, Bayley, Michel, & Pugh, 1986, p. 55).

In addition, the ethics committee should evaluate its own work on a routine basis. This should involve a review of the purpose and functions of the committee by committee members. The committee can also check with home care personnel to see if the committee is making their work harder or easier. The committee members must strive to keep involved in the mainstream of the home care provider's work and not isolate themselves from practical concerns.

Though ethics committees will not be able to resolve all ethical problems that arise in home care, they are an important forum for the discussion of an increasing number of perplexing issues. The ethics committee is in a prime position to identify the ethical issues (as opposed to the emotional, clinical, and legal ones) and spell out the conflicting values involved in individual cases or in policies.

SUMMARY

Ethical decision making is never easy, but it is especially challenging on an organizational level. Methods that have been helpful in resolving ethical problems and clarifying organizational values have been provided. Codes of ethics can provide minimal practice standards and a guide for administrators and employees. Ethics committees can serve as a valuable resource in the decision-making process.

Commitment to ethical ideals should arise from within the home care organization from its commitment to a philosophy of care and regard for the dignity of the individuals and families it serves. The impetus for formal work in ethics, such as policy development, can arise from the "grass-roots" level or from top-level administrators. In either case, the support and commitment of the top-level executive is essential to the survival of ethical practice. Without this level of commitment, home care personnel, especially direct caregivers, will not be confident of the administrative support to make ethically sound decisions. The tools presented in this chapter can improve the quality of ethical decisions by staff and administration by providing them with guidelines to analyze an ethical problem and the support to choose the best course of action.

REFERENCES

American Academy of Pediatrics, Committee on Bioethics. (1983). Treatment of critically ill newborns. *Pediatrics, 72*(4): 565–566.

American Hospital Association. (1972). *A Patient's Bill of Rights.* Chicago: American Hospital Publishing, Inc.

American Medical Association Council Report. (1985). Guidelines for ethics committees in health care institutions. *Journal of the American Medical Association, 253*(18): 2698–2699.

American Nurses' Association. (1986). *Standards of Home Health Nursing Practice.* Kansas City, Mo: American Nurses' Association.

Annas, G.J. (1984). Ethics committees in neonatal care: Substantive protection or procedural diversion? *American Journal of Public Health, 74*(8): 843–845.

Baginski, Y. (1989). Pediatric bioethics: A community-based committee's experience. *Caring, 8*(3): 14–19.

Bayley, C. (1986). The inner life of an ethics committee. *Hospital Ethics, 2*(6): 5–6.

Berney, K. (1987). Finding the ethical edge. *Nation's Business, 75*(8): 18–24.

Drane J.F., & Roth, R.B. (1985). Institutional ethics committees: What, how, and why. *Health Progress, 66*(8): 30–34, 56.

Gaylin, W. (1973). The patient' bill of rights. *Saturday Review of the Sciences, 1*(2): 22.

Glaser, J. (1989, October). *Biomedical ethics: An overview.* Paper presented at the Intensive Ethics Seminar for Pharmacy Faculty, Omaha, Neb.

Heron, E. (1987). *Intensive Care Nurse.* New York: Ivy Books.

In re Quinlan, 70 NJ 10, 355 A2d 647 (1976).

Jaret, P. (1984). The final guardians. *Newsweek*, 104(24):16.

Joint Commission on Accreditation of Healthcare Organizations. (1988). *Standards for Accreditation of Home Care.* Chicago: Joint Commission on Accreditation of Healthcare Organizations.

Levine, C. (1984). Questions and (some very tenative) answers about hospital ethics committees. *Hastings Center Report, 14*(3): 9–12.

Lowy, L. (1979). *Social Work with the Aging.* New York: Harper & Row.

Macklin, R., & Kupfer, R.B. (1988). *Hospital Ethics Committees: Manual for a Training Program.* New York: Albert Einstein College of Medicine.

McCarrick, P.M., & Adams, J. (1987). *Ethics committees in Hospitals* (Scope Note 3). Washington, DC: Georgetown University, Kennedy Institute of Ethics.

O'Rourke, K.D., & Brodeur, D. (1989). *Medical Ethics: Common Ground for Understanding.* St. Louis: The Catholic Health Association.

Peters, T.J., & Waterman, R.H. (1982). *In Search of Excellence.* New York: Harper & Row.

Ross, J.W., Bayley, C., Michel, V., & Pugh, D. (1986). *Handbook for Hospital Ethics Committees.* Chicago: American Hospital Publishing, Inc.

Thompson, J.E., & Thompson, H.O. (1985). *Bioethical Decision Making for Nurses*. Norwalk, Conn: Appleton-Century-Crofts.

Ufema, J. (1984). Personal concerns of the hospice movement. *American Journal of Hospice Care*, *1*(1): 5–6.

Young, A., Pignatello, C.H., & Taylor, M.B. (1988). Who's the boss? Ethical conflicts in home care. *Health Progress*, *69*(11): 59–62.

Index